T0324234

Journeys in
Medicine and Research
on Three Continents
Over 50 Years

Journeys in
Medicine and Research on Three Continents Over 50 Years

Moyra Smith
University of California, Irvine, USA

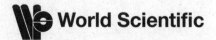

World Scientific

NEW JERSEY · LONDON · SINGAPORE · BEIJING · SHANGHAI · HONG KONG · TAIPEI · CHENNAI · TOKYO

Published by

World Scientific Publishing Co. Pte. Ltd.
5 Toh Tuck Link, Singapore 596224
USA office: 27 Warren Street, Suite 401-402, Hackensack, NJ 07601
UK office: 57 Shelton Street, Covent Garden, London WC2H 9HE

Library of Congress Cataloging-in-Publication Data
Names: Smith, Moyra, author.
Title: Journeys in medicine and research on three continents over 50 years / Moyra Smith.
Description: New Jersey : World Scientific, 2017. |
   Includes bibliographical references and index.
Identifiers: LCCN 2017021818| ISBN 9789813209534 (hardcover : alk. paper) |
   ISBN 9813209534 (hardcover : alk. paper) | ISBN 9789813209541 (pbk. : alk. paper) |
   ISBN 9813209542 (pbk. : alk. paper)
Subjects: | MESH: Medicine--trends | Socioeconomic Factors | Communicable Diseases |
   Genetic Diseases, Inborn | Personal Narratives
Classification: LCC RA418 | NLM WB 100 | DDC 362.1--dc23
LC record available at https://lccn.loc.gov/2017021818

British Library Cataloguing-in-Publication Data
A catalogue record for this book is available from the British Library.

Printed in Singapore

This work is dedicated to family, friends, mentors, colleagues, students and patients who inspired me throughout my journeys

Epigraph

"Scientists therefore are used to dealing with doubt and uncertainty.
I believe that to solve any problem .... you have to permit the possibility
that you do not have it exactly right." Richard Feynman

Preface

This book is designed for an audience with interest in health and societal factors. It is in part autobiographical, based on different phases of my life in Medicine over 50 years. I revisit cases and problems encountered as I worked in different countries, including South Africa, Scotland, England and North America. Essays encompass aspects of clinical medicine and aspects of research, particularly in Genetics and Genomic Medicine.

In each section I discuss situations and clinical problems that I confronted in the past and in addition, I review new information on the topic or disorder and current opinions and approaches to finding solutions. In a number of sections, I review aspects of the history of development of pertinent ideas.

Perhaps this book is a hybrid, the subject matter lies between medical sciences, social sciences and philosophy.

An underlying philosophical question has to do with the degree to which we, as physicians, and scientists, are able to deal with changes and also with partial fixes of problems. For many physicians and researchers, in the modern era especially, we are driven to find the root causes of specific diseases with the hope that discovery of root causes can lead to more effective treatment and possibly even to disease elimination. We are fortunate that science and technology in the 20th and 21st century furnish us with inspiring examples of situations where discovery of underlying causes of disease led to discovery of solutions. We are, however, also confronted by many examples of diseases where root causes are complex and where we have to make do with partial fixes and symptom reduction. In addition, as healthcare workers, we need to confront the realities of disease causation linked to socioeconomic and political and conflict situations that seem impossible to resolve.

Contents

Acknowledgements

I wish to thank World Scientific Publishing Editor Sook Cheng Lim and co-editors for their work on this book. I am grateful for access to the University of California library and Internet resources. I particularly acknowledge observers, researchers and authors whose efforts have led to progress in the life sciences over the past 50 years.

PART I

Social Dimensions of Health

1 Looking Back

At this distance in miles, and in time (more than seventy years) what images arise as I think of South Africa? There are vistas of open veldt, grassy plains with occasional flat-topped thorn trees and blue mountains at the edge of the horizon. There are images of wild flowers, aloes with fleshy leaves and orange, red and yellow blossoms on tall erect stems.

In my memories there are dark-skinned people who walk erect as they carry objects on their heads. There are women with elaborate head-wraps; sometimes they wear many necklaces. There are men and women who in winter drape themselves with colorful blankets with geometric designs. Women sing songs with words I do not understand, yet they move me.

I remember the African sunrise. At one moment, the earth was dark and at the next, bright orange rays illuminated the whole sky.

During high summer on the veldt we could see the air shimmer at midday. The heat was heavy, tangible. Once on the Highveld, when the rains came after a long period of drought we children, black and white, ran outside to lift our faces to the sky and feel the drenching moisture on our hot skins.

Once, as I watched the sun setting beyond fields and fields of maize, the sky was filled with reds and yellows and the moon rose as a giant disc.

As I remember the beauty of South Africa, I think of family and gardens. My mother loved flowers and shrubs and spent many hours working in the garden. I recall working alongside Mom and her helper James, when I was about eight years old. James dug the earth, Mom placed the plants and together we pressed the earth firmly around them.

Who was James? A few years after the war perhaps around 1946–1947 a young black man came to the door to ask my mother if she had work for him. He told her he had come on the train to Johannesburg from the countryside. He had then walked far looking unsuccessfully for work and had spent all his money. My mother decided to give James work. I believe James was about sixteen years old when he came to our household.

Houses in Johannesburg frequently had a room and a bathroom in the backyard. We used the room as a playroom. When James came my mother instructed us to remove all our toys from the backroom, this was now to be James' room.

James helped with chores in the house and garden. My mother helped James improve his skills at reading and writing and arithmetic. She and James opened a savings account for him at the local post-office. Mom and James kept a tally of the accumulating funds. I remember the happy day when James realized he had saved enough money to buy a bicycle!

At one point during his stay with us, James became very ill. Mom was very worried, we had no car to drive him to the hospital. She called around to find a doctor who would make a house call and so it was that we got to meet Doctor Jean Donne. She was an imposing but friendly Scots woman. She arrived at our home wearing a woolen suit and matching felt hat. My mother and Doctor Donne went into James' room and my sister and I waited outside. Dr. Donne examined James and determined that he needed to be hospitalized because he had pneumonia. She called for an ambulance and waited with him until the ambulance arrived. My sister and I watched tearfully as James was moved onto a stretcher and carried to the ambulance.

After a long while, perhaps only a few weeks, James came home again. He had a follow-up appointment at Dr. Donne's office. He told us that she was a very kind doctor.

A few years later James told us that now he was a grown-up man and he should not work in the house but should find other work, so he left with our good wishes.

During the first seven years of my childhood I spent many months as a patient in hospital. It was this experience that fueled my ambition to become a doctor. During the years when I was a patient I never met a female physician. It was my encounter with Dr. Donne that led me to think it was possible to become a doctor.

The Witwatersrand and Mining

I was raised in Johannesburg, South Africa. The mine dumps were prominent features of the landscape. These dumps were pale yellow in color and they contained the material that remained after the ore-bearing rock was crushed and chemically treated to extract gold. On windy days, light yellow dust originated from the newer mines, would be blown around the southern suburbs of the city and the atmosphere was hazy with fine particles. On older mines the yellow sand had been compacted down to the consistency of soft rock that was subject to erosion when the rains came. The land around the mine dumps was bare. Nothing grew in the soil that was laden with chemicals.

Pneumoconiosis was one of the difficult yet intriguing words I learned in childhood. I first saw the word as my mother and I travelled on a bus. The word appeared on one of the large buildings near the city center. The sign read "Pneumoconiosis Bureau, Chamber of Mines". My mother explained that pneumoconiosis was the word used to explain the chronic cough of men who worked in the mines, men who seemed weak though they were not yet old.

As children we learned that the mineshafts in the area around Johannesburg, the Witwatersrand, were the deepest in the world. It seemed as though the men went down to the great depths in the mines where their lungs became filled with some of the same dust and debris that made the mine dumps.

Some years later when I was in high school we watched a newsreel about a breakthrough in mining technology. The silica dust present in the mines, generated by drilling rock, was reduced when drills were attached to high pressure water sprays. It was difficult to imagine where all that water could come from to supply the high pressure drills, given the relatively low rainfall in the area and the frequent droughts that occurred. The mining companies were allowed to tap into the gold and into underground water streams.

Political Tensions

I remember the tumultuous political events that occurred in South Africa when I was in high school and when I was a medical student. Problems related to inequality and segregation had been festering for many decades. The situation became particularly intense and disturbing in the 1950's.

I have a memory from my early high school years, perhaps before 1953, of standing with my mother on a sidewalk in the central city in Johannesburg where we had gone to take care of business. We watched large open-backed trucks drive by. Standing in the back of the trucks were black men and women. They were singing stirring songs. The trucks drove by slowly and at one point a truck filled with black women stopped alongside us. My mother told me that these people had been demonstrating against "the system". They had been arrested and were being driven to Marshall Square, the central police station. I felt a chill run through me. We all feared the police. On the opposite side of the street from us white women stood side by side in a long line, each woman wore a wide Black Sash draped from her right shoulder to her waist. These white women stood silently demonstrating against the apartheid system and against loss of freedom. My mother remarked how courageous they were.

2 Socio-economic Factors and Health: Medical School and Beyond

My ambitions to become a doctor were further fueled during my years in high school by the many books I read, including Paul de Kruif's *Microbe Hunters,* and the biography of Harvey Cushing, neurosurgeon. I read novels by A.J. Cronin and Axel Munthe; both of these authors were physicians and their novels portrayed the struggles and joys of being a physician.

My years in medical school were filled with hard work, studying hard to keep my scholarship and working in the vacations to earn money for books. I must confess I was only partly aware of political changes and crises. My family was deeply disturbed by the killing of demonstrators at Sharpeville in 1960. I felt a sense of hopelessness. My mother encouraged me to concentrate on my studies. And so, for the next three years, I continued to concentrate on my studies and on my work in the clinics and hospital wards.

As a medical student and later as an intern and junior physician working in South Africa questions relating to socio-economic factors and their impact on health frequently came to mind.

In the 1960s on the pediatric wards in South Africa one frequently encountered little patients with problems seldom seen in Europe or North America. Kwashiorkor was common among South African black children. Kwashiorkor is a word from Ghana which means "the displaced one" and is derived from the observation that signs of this disorder commonly developed when breast feeding of that child ceased, perhaps the mother's milk had dried up or a new child was born. Children in the early stages of kwashiorkor showed changes in hair color, the black hair took on a reddish hue. Later, the affected child's belly swelled and the child became progressively more withdrawn. In the severest cases of kwashiorkor, the hands and feet swelled, skin blistered and peeled. Liver, kidney and brain were progressively damaged. Prevention was simple, protein in diet needed to be increased. As a medical student I remember talking with a mother who was about to take home her two-year-old child who had recently recovered from kwashiorkor. I explained to her that to prevent a recurrence of the illness she should feed the child more protein rich food, milk, meat. She lowered her head and told me about her life. She and her mother lived in one room of a house in the township located about 10 miles from the city. Each weekday she travelled to the city to do laundry In private homes. A large percentage of her income was spent on paying rent for the room. Much of the remainder was spent on bus fares to and from the city to the township. The child's father had moved to another city to find work and he did not send money to support them. Corn meal was the only food they could regularly afford. As I listened to her story, I felt saddened and outraged that a women worked each day, lived in one room and was not paid enough to support adequate nutrition. The best I could do was to give her a month's supply of milk powder and to schedule a follow-up visit for mother and child when more milk powder could be supplied.

Rescuing a few infants from the devastating complications of protein malnutrition was satisfying if one did not stop to think of the untended cases and if one did not think that rescue might be only temporary.

When I worked as an intern on the Gynecology service at the general hospital in Pretoria I frequently took care of young African women who were admitted because of severe vaginal bleeding. Often they had high fevers and had lost large quantities of blood. These desperately ill women would say very little. It was only when we examined them that we realized that their breasts were full and that they had probably been pregnant. They had miscarried. We did not know whether the miscarriage was spontaneous or induced. Their treatment included blood transfusion, antibiotics and curettage of the uterus to remove remaining partial products of conception. The women stayed in the hospital until they were well. We did not discuss the danger of back-room abortion with them. Perhaps there was no need, they had already experienced the consequences.

In the 1960s, medical contraception was just becoming an option in South Africa. For low wage earners it was an expensive option and the law required the signature of a spouse before a woman could be given a prescription for contraception.

3 Trauma and Experiences in the Surgical Unit at Baragwanath

After graduating from medical school in 1963 I took a position as an intern in surgery at Baragwanath Hospital, which served the people of Soweto. South Africa was racially segregated at the time and Soweto was a sprawling suburb for "non-whites" located about forty miles from Johannesburg. Soweto accommodated many people who had come from rural areas to find work in the city. Housing was for the most part inadequate. The streets were poorly lit and the roads were dusty tracks. Entertainment and sports facilities were almost non-existent then. Beer parlors "shebeens", where a potent home-brewed beer was sold, were plentiful. Particularly at the end of each month when workers were paid, gang members accosted them on their way home and frequently used violent methods to relieve workers of their meager earnings.

People from Soweto who worked in Johannesburg travelled to and from work by train. Trains were infrequent and they were usually over-crowded. Passengers who could not find a place in the cars held onto posts at the entrance of the cars and it often seemed as though they barely had a foothold on the steps. This situation often led to accidents.

Baragwanath Hospital was established in a large complex of separated single story buildings that had been constructed as army barracks during the Second World War. These buildings housed the patient wards, the laboratories, hospital service facilities and the interns' residence.

A surgical internship at Bara, as we called the hospital, was a very intense experience. There were many trauma cases and the patient to physician ratio was very high. At the end of the month and at weekends and on public holidays the alcohol intake and the crime rate in Soweto rose steeply and the surgical wards at Bara were overflowing. After a heavy patient intake all the hospital beds were filled and patients occupied cots between the beds and down the central aisle of the large wards.

We worked as a team, junior and senior doctors and nurses. Bara represented the best team experience of my life. The pace was very fast, there was no room for egos and competition. We all needed to do the best we could and as efficiently as possible.

One part of the team was in the operating room (OR), the other part of the team remained in the ward on intake. Urgent trauma cases by-passed the emergency room and were brought directly to the ward. Often, several severely wounded patients would arrive simultaneously, and there was a split second decision to make on whom to treat first. Stab wounds to the chest, neck or abdomen were most the common. These included stabbed heart, stabbed arteries, stabbed lung. If the stab wound maintained an open passage to the outside the lung often collapsed. This was less of a problem than when the outer wound sealed and the stabbed lung leaked air into the pleural cavity, leading to pneumothorax. Air in the pleural cavity could lead to compression of the central structures in the chest, to major arteries and veins, and to compression of the heart.

Patients with stab wounds had frequently hemorrhaged severely and they arrived in shock; sometimes they lay still, sometimes they were restless and agitated. I remember when David, a man in his early twenties, was rushed into the unit. "Stabbed carotid artery" the orderly said. I looked up to see the rest of the surgical team just exiting from the far end of the ward hurrying to the OR for an urgent surgery. I needed to start managing the case immediately without them. He lay still, which was fortunate since there was a clot plugging the wound which could have readily dislodged if he moved. There were no veins visible and his pulse was very weak, signs that he had bled profusely. A nurse rushed over with the infusion set and the cut down equipment and I cut down carefully into the surface tissues of the right wrist above the thumb. This is a position where there is usually a large vein. As the nurse shone a flashlight onto the incision, I was able to see a pale vein and I inserted a catheter. We obtained a blood sample for typing and cross match for blood transfusion and we began to pump in plasma. We had pumped in 5 units of plasma, almost 2 liters, before the pulse strengthened. We sent a message to the surgical team that we were rushing a patient to the OR, for surgical repair of a left carotid artery.

David recovered, but was left with a moderate weakness on the right side of his body. He was puzzled that his right side was weak since the stab wound was on the left side of the neck. We explained that the brain tissue on the left side of his brain suffered the worst oxygen deprivation. Since major nerves originating on the left side of the brain cross over to the right before they enter the spinal cord, he experienced weakness on the right.

Lazarus, a man in his twenties, was brought by ambulance to the surgical ward directly from the train station. He arrived in the early morning when most members of our team were performing surgery on non-emergency "cold" cases and my back-up intern was in the out-patient clinic. Lazarus was one of the people hanging from the posts at the entrance of the train when the train jerked. He fell off and under the train; as the train moved on his legs were amputated. Tourniquets had been placed on the stumps to stop the bleeding, but not before he had sustained significant blood loss. He arrived at the ward in shock and restless and calling out "Where are my legs?". A nurse assisted me as cautious sedation was continued, and a cut down was done to gain access to a vein, to pump in plasma to begin to restore circulation volume before the matched blood arrived for infusion. Lazarus was then taken to the OR and the surgical team spent many hours repairing torn vessels, removing damaged tissue and creating functional stumps that could later accommodate artificial limbs.

I remember being at his bedside on the second day after surgery when Lazarus drowsily looked up at the intravenous fluid container and said, "I make those". He worked for a medical supply company and was on his way to work when he fell from the train.

After a few weeks, Lazarus could place himself in a wheelchair and he left our ward for the rehabilitation unit at Bara. From time to time I would meet him as he vigorously propelled his wheelchair along the outdoor passage ways and paths. He was full of energy and determined to overcome his difficulties. Later he was fitted with artificial limbs.

The Christmas season at Bara was a nightmare, more trauma and more patients. The fact that beer flowed more freely likely played a role. Our team took over from one of the other surgical teams on Christmas Day and then we worked for two days and nights with very little rest. On the morning of the third day after Christmas our chief told us it was really important to discharge all patients that could safely be let go. The overcrowding had reached intolerable proportions and New Year's Eve and holiday were rapidly approaching. Michael, a man in his early thirties, was one of the patients whom the chief thought could be discharged. He had a stab wound to the chest. The wound was deep, however chest X-ray on admission and on the second day indicated that there was no air in the pleural cavity. Patients were scheduled to leave by early evening. After completing tasks in the ward I went to my room, collapsed on the bed and fell immediately asleep. Before long, the insistent ringing of the telephone woke me. It was the senior nurse. "When Michael started to move around to dress and leave he didn't feel well and he asked if he might stay longer". "Yes, please keep him there, I will be right over", I replied. When I examined Michael I found that the breath sounds on the side of the stab wound were now muffled. A chest X-ray revealed air in the pleural cavity. The most likely explanation for his changed condition was that the wound in the lung had sealed with a blood clot which dislodged as he moved around. I inserted a needle, connected tubing and a vacuum unit to drain the air. Michael felt more comfortable almost immediately. Thank goodness he had asked to stay. He might have died at home. We contained drainage for a day and then carefully monitored Michael as he resumed physical activity to try to be sure it was safe for him to be discharged.

Two weeks later I saw Michael in the out-patient clinic. He was well, active and back at work. As he was leaving the clinic he handed me a gift, a recording of folk-songs. Michael said he was grateful to me for letting him stay longer in the hospital. I thanked him but omitted that we were grateful to him for saving us from the consequences of an error in judgement.

Mark was a patient in his late twenties who arrived in the unit at about 2 a.m. He had been stabbed in the back and the knife was still in his back. His blood pressure was only slightly elevated and his neurological examination was normal. He lay face down on the examining table and he yelled, "Get the knife out!" As he yelled, the small examining room filled with alcohol fumes.

We had been taught that one should never impulsively remove a weapon such as a knife. One needed to assess where the knife was located relative to important body structures. I explained to Mark that we needed to get X-ray studies to examine the positon of the knife and I gave him medication for the pain. The X-ray studies were done fairly promptly. His anger raged on throughout despite the pain medication. "What kind of a place is this? A man has a knife in his back and you leave it there!" I reviewed the X-rays with the radiologist. It seemed that the knife was firmly embedded in the body of a vertebra; fortunately, the tip of the knife had not penetrated to the canal through which the spinal cord runs.

I hurried to the OR to explain the situation to the rest of the team and to request permission to remove the knife since I knew they would be tied for several hours on emergency surgery on other patients. "Bring him to the treatment room adjacent to the OR and go ahead and remove the knife, we will be close by in case there are complications", the chief surgeon said. A nurse and I wheeled the trolley with the cussing patient to the treatment room. I injected the tissues around the knife with a local anesthetic and when it had taken effect I tried to pull the knife out. It would not budge. I am physically quite small and I wondered if I would fail to carry out the treatment. I then asked the nurse to stand behind me and I placed my right foot behind me in a horizontal position and asked her to brace her foot against mine. I pulled mightily and slowly the weapon came out. The nurse saved me from falling over backward. "Why didn't you do that long ago?" the patient yelled. There was no excessive bleeding. We monitored Mark for infection and fortunately there were no neurological complications.

It was late at night, after the acute emergencies had been dealt with, that I got to examine Mr. M., a man in his fifties, who had been admitted because of chest pain after an episode of vomiting. Mr. M. was not restless, he lay quietly and did not complain. As I placed a stethoscope on his chest to listen to his heart and breath sounds it seemed as though small bubbles were moving away as the skin and underlying tissues were gently compressed. I then palpated the chest wall and again there was the same strange sensation; it seemed as though I was compressing a sponge. As I puzzled over this I remembered a paragraph that I had read in a surgery textbook, which described the case of a famous admiral of the Dutch fleet who was accustoming to indulging in large feasts. After one such feast he became ill and in the process of throwing up he had ruptured his esophagus. The author of the textbook noted that one of the signs of a ruptured esophagus is "crepitus" of the chest wall. Crepitus was described as a crackling sensation as one compresses the soft tissues of the chest wall. Air passes through the tear in the esophagus into the surrounding tissue sand then into the chest wall and gives rise to crepitus. Ruptured esophagus is a dangerous condition, in part because accumulation of air in the tissues surrounding the esophagus and central structures of the chest can lead to compression of the great blood vessels and impede blood flow. Leakage of fluid from a tear in the esophagus also leads to infection in the adjacent tissues.

I concluded that Mr. M. most likely had a ruptured esophagus and rushed to the OR to inform the senior surgeon on our team. He was somewhat disbelieving of my diagnosis (particularly since I was the most junior member on the team), but he recommended that I alert the radiologist immediately and recommend a swallowing study with a small quantity of a solution containing a dye that could be visualized in X-ray. The swallowing study and X-ray demonstrated that dye tracked out of the esophagus into the surrounding tissue.

Mr. M. underwent surgery to repair the tear in his esophagus. Following vigorous antibiotic therapy, he recovered. I felt very grateful to the author of the textbook for including the anecdote about the admiral, without this I might not have remembered the significance of chest wall crepitus.

Mr. M. and I both had a lucky break. I had delayed seeing him while taking care of other cases. Despite his composure his condition was dangerous and he should have been higher on my list of priorities. I realized that assessment of a patient's status depends in part on communication. Patients who suffer bravely and silently often present the greatest challenge.

Esophageal Cancer

The surgical unit to which I was assigned at Baragwanath Hospital in Soweto provided services to patients with many different types of surgical problems. In addition to coping with trauma patients, the chief of the unit specialized in esophageal surgery and all patients admitted to the hospital who had evidence of esophageal problems were assigned to our unit. In talking with those patients I learned that many of them were resident in an eastern region of South Africa referred to as the Transkei and they had travelled considerable distances in search of treatments. I wondered if specific environmental risk factors existed in that region contributed to development of esophageal cancer. These patients presented with difficulties in swallowing and with severe weight loss. Various procedures were carried out to improve their nutritional status; these included insertion of feeding tubes. In some cases, surgeries were carried out to remove the cancerous lesions that were located primarily in the upper two-thirds of the esophagus and the cancer was found to be of the squamous cell type. Despite treatments, the outlook for these patients was bleak.

Recently I reviewed the occurrence of esophageal cancer in different regions of the world, the different types of cancer that occur and information on likely risk factors. Squamous carcinoma occurs primarily in the upper two-thirds of the esophagus; adenocarcinoma occurs in the lower third of the esophagus. In Europe, squamous carcinoma and adenocarcinoma of the esophagus occur with equal frequency. In many other regions of the world the squamous form of esophageal cancer predominates and the incidence of this form is particularly high in Turkey, Iran, Kazakhstan and in southern and eastern regions of Africa, (Pennathur *et al.*, 2013). In a report from South Africa, Cotton *et al.* (2014) noted that esophageal cancer still impacts many people in the Transkei region of South Africa and is the leading cause of cancer deaths in males and the second highest cause of cancer deaths in women.

Fumonisin exposure has been linked to the pathogenesis of esophageal cancer. Shephard *et al.* (2007) compared fumonisin intake in individuals in two areas of South Africa. In one area fumonisin intake was low and esophageal cancer incidence was low, in a second area fumonisin intake was high and the incidence of esophageal cancer was high. Shepard *et al.* reported that in the area with high incidence of esophageal cancer the daily intake was double that found in individuals in low esophageal cancer risk area. Fumonisin intake was also demonstrated to be high in regions of Iran where the esophageal cancer incidence was high (Shephard *et al.*, 2002). A number of studies have proposed that contamination of foods, particularly maize, with molds that produce fumonisin toxins constitute an important risk factor. However, the importance of fumonisin in esophageal cancer etiology is not widely accepted.

Other widely accepted risk factors contributing to esophageal cancer include tobacco and alcohol use, poor nutrition with inadequate vitamin intake and poor oral hygiene (Cotton *et al.*, 2014).

South Africa in the Past and in the Present Millennium

In a comprehensive paper on "Urbanization and Development in South Africa", Ivan Turok (2012) noted:

> "For over a century urbanization has been a source of controversy, posing dilemmas for successive governments resulting in wide ranging intervention to control it in various ways".

Turok noted further that in the mid-20th century particularly draconian controls were imposed. These control became known as "apartheid".

Turok traced the history of problems related to urbanization, migration, inadequate housing and racial discrimination. He noted that many of these problems began in the late 19th and the early 20th centuries following discovery of diamonds near Kimberley in 1867 and gold in the Witwatersrand in 1884. Mining required intense labor. The mining companies recruited black South African men from rural areas. These men were hired with temporary contracts. They were accommodated in dormitories without their families. In addition, South African mining companies encouraged influx of temporary workers from other African states, including Mozambique to the East and states to the North.

Statistics revealed that by 1910 the number of single black men accommodated in mining dormitories exceeded 100,000 and their number increased steadily thereafter. He noted that the "mining revolution" had profound effects on social relations and racial discrimination.

The closed accommodation for mine workers facilitated the spread of diseases. Furthermore, as temporary migrant workers subsequently returned to their families in rural areas they transmitted their diseases to their families. Packard (1989) reported that by the late 1920's significant number of adults in the rural Transkei and Ciskei regions of South Africa were infected with tuberculosis.

Turok noted that as additional industries grew up around major cities in South Africa, specific urban municipalities began to provide housing in townships for black families. Increasingly these townships were primarily located at the periphery of urban areas. Transport into the cities for work was complicated and relatively expensive for workers, given the wages they earned.

The post-apartheid history of South Africa began in 1994 with the election of Nelson Mandela as president and then the country faced considerable challenges with optimism.

Turok emphasized that in post-apartheid South Africa "poverty traps" still existed on the periphery of major cities. He noted that economic growth has lagged behind population growth.

In the period between 1999 and 2008 significant damage to population health resulted from governmental health policies that under-estimated the HIV-AIDS epidemic and denied the use of scientific principles in its treatment.

In 2009, Coovadia et al. authored a significant paper, "The health and the health system in South Africa" that was published in the Lancet medical journal. In assessing the impact of relative diseases they used the DALY measure. The disability-adjusted life year (DALY) is a measure of overall disease burden, expressed as the number of years lost due to ill-health, disability or early death. Coovadia et al. noted that HIV-AIDS was the prime disease factor and resulted in 31% of the total disability adjusted years (DALYS) in the South African population. Interpersonal violence was the next highest factor (DALY 6.5%). Tuberculosis accounted for 3.7%; road traffic injuries accounted for 3.0% of the DALY and diarrheal infection accounted for 2.9%.

In 2012, Mayosi et al. published a follow-up Lancet paper, "Health in South Africa changes and challenges since 2009". They reported that HIV-AIDS and tuberculosis were the most significant problems in South Africa. South Africa had the largest anti-retroviral administration program in the world with 1.8 million people taking anti-retroviral medications. They noted that the tuberculosis epidemic continued unabated; however, there were hopes that revised and improved rapid testing for drug resistant Mycobacterium tuberculosis strains would yield progress in early diagnosis and treatment.

Mayosi *et al.* reported that there were some indications that mortality from inter-personal violence and traffic accidents had slightly decreased. However, the incidence of violence against women had not decreased.

The report concluded that in 2011 South Africa was not on track with progress toward a number of the Millennium Development Goals set by the World Health Organization (www.who.int/mdg/en/), but it had potential to advance toward those goals.

WHO Millennium Development Goals (MDG)

MDG1: Eradicate extreme poverty and hunger.
MDG2: Achieve universal primary education.
MDG3: Promote gender equality and empower women.
MDG4: Reduce child mortality by two thirds from 1990 levels.
MDG5: Improve maternal health, reduce the 1990 maternal mortality rate by three quarters.
MDG6: Combat HIV-AIDS, malaria and other infectious diseases.

References

Coovadia H, Jewkes R, Barron P, *et al.* (2009). The health and health system of South Africa: historical roots of current public health challenges. *Lancet* **374(9692):**817–34. doi: 10.1016/S0140-6736(09)60951-X. PMID:19709728.

Cotton RG, Langer R, Leong T, *et al.* (2014). Coping with esophageal cancer approaches worldwide. *Ann N Y Acad Sci* **1325:**138–58. doi: 10.1111/nyas.12522. PMID:25266022.

Mayosi BM, Lawn JE, van Niekerk A, *et al.* (2012). Health in South Africa: changes and challenges since 2009. *Lancet* **380(9858):**2029–43. doi: 10.1016/S0140-6736(12)61814-5. PMID:23201214.

Packard RM. (1989). *White plague, Black Labor Tuberculosis and the Political Economy of Health and Disease in South Africa.* University of California Press.

Pennathur A, Gibson MK, Jobe BA, Luketich JD. (2013). Oesophageal carcinoma. *Lancet* **381(9864):**400–12. doi: 10.1016/S0140-6736(12)60643-6. PMID:23374478.

Shephard GS, Marasas WF, Yazdanpanah H, *et al.* (2002). Fumonisin B(1) in maize harvested in Iran during 1999. *Food Addit Contam* **19(7):**676–9. PMID:12113663

Shephard GS, Marasas WF, Burger HM, *et al.* (2007). Exposure assessment for fumonisins in the former Transkei region of South Africa. *Food Addit Contam* **24(6):**621–9. PMID:17487603.

Smith, Moyra. Parts of the material presented in 'South Africa: Land of beauty and despair' were included in an MFA thesis presented at Antioch University.

Turok I. (2012). Urbanisation and Development in South Africa: Economic Imperatives, Spatial Distortions and Strategic Responses. International Institute for Environment and Development, United Nations Population Fund working paper 10621.

PART II

Mothers and Children

5 Pregnancy and Hazards

There are two particular cases that are still embedded in my memories of time spent as an intern in Obstetrics in South Africa in 1964. Both cases came in as patients to a small mission hospital located at some distance from Pretoria.

One case involved a pregnant woman brought into the hospital by her frantic husband. She had been having seizures and was only partly conscious. This woman had no prior history of seizures. The diagnosis in this patient was eclampsia, a very serious condition that can lead to death.

The second patient, Mrs. X., was a middle-aged woman who was admitted to the hospital on a very busy Saturday afternoon when several patients in advanced labor were admitted at about the same time. I was not present when Mrs. X. delivered; one of the nuns assisted in the delivery. When I arrived a little later at Mrs. X's side, the sister told me that she had delivered a stillborn infant and that the placenta had also been delivered. This was Mrs. X.'s twelfth delivery. The sister was anxious to transfer Mrs. X. to the general ward to make room in the labor ward for other patients. Mrs. X. seemed very distressed and weak to me and I asked the sister to delay transfer until I had examined this patient. As I pulled back the sheets I realized that Mrs. X. was hemorrhaging profusely. On internal examination there was evidence of uterine rupture. I called for help to summon an obstetric surgeon and an anesthetist and I began blood transfusions, eventually using the entire group O Rh negative blood available at the small hospital and the transfusing plasma. I tried other measures including packing with bandages. Tragically, Mrs. X. died before the surgeon arrived.

These cases have remained vividly in my mind and conscience. Now, more than 50 years later, I returned to the literature to examine newer information on the causes of eclampsia and ruptured uterus and their frequencies in different regions of the world.

Pre-eclampsia and Eclampsia

Pre-eclampsia occurs world-wide and is reported to impact 3–5% of pregnancies (www.pre-eclampsia.org). Symptoms of pre-eclampsia usually manifest after the 20th week of pregnancy. The key initial manifestations are raised blood pressure (blood pressure higher than 140 systolic and 90 diastolic), and increased amounts of protein excretion in the urine, more than 300 mg of protein in a 24-hour urine collection. The degree of proteinuria varies in different patients. Swelling (edema) was previously considered to be a manifestation of pre-eclampsia. However, swelling is now not considered to be a key pre-eclampsia manifestation since it is common in late pregnancy in women who do not have increased blood pressure.

The placenta plays a key role in the pathogenesis of pre-eclampsia (Young et al., 2010). The fact that pre-eclampsia can occur in situations where placental-like tissue accumulations (hydatiform mole) occur in the absence of a fetus proves that it is the placenta that leads to pre-eclampsia.

Pre-eclampsia occurs more commonly in young women during their first pregnancy. It also occurs more commonly in multi-fetus pregnancies and in women who have other chronic health conditions, including diabetes. Advanced maternal age is also a risk factor for pre-eclampsia.

In situations where access to healthcare is limited, pre-eclampsia can go on to become a severe systemic disease, eclampsia. Severe progressive consequences of pre-eclampsia are signaled by occurrence of headaches, blurred vision and/or tight-sided abdominal upper quadrant pain due to liver involvement, and decreased urine production that may progress to renal failure. In some cases, hematologic manifestations may occur. These include breakdown of red blood cells (hemolysis) and an abnormally low platelet count (thrombocytopenia). Hemolysis, elevated liver enzymes and low platelet count have been designated as a defined syndrome, the HELPP syndrome. In the severest, the brain may be affected and seizures and loss of consciousness occurs. In women with eclampsia the fetus and placenta must be rapidly delivered to prevent maternal death.

In developed countries, eclampsia is rare and the main complications of pre-eclampsia center around early delivery of the fetus and placenta to prevent severe complications of pre-eclampsia, including eclampsia. Early delivery of the fetus may lead to complications of prematurity. In developing countries maternal deaths from severe forms of pre-eclampsia and eclampsia occur and worldwide these are estimated to reach 60,000.

Young *et al.* (2010) reported evidence that in pre-eclampsia increased amounts of specific anti-angiogenic factors are present in the maternal circulation. These anti-angiogenic factors include a specific factor, soluble FMs-like tyrosine kinase, that inhibits blood vessel growth and specifically binds to vascular endothelial growth factor (VEGF). Another anti-angiogenic factor that is increased in the circulation in pre-eclampsia is soluble endoglin. These anti-angiogenic factors damage the endothelial cells of blood vessels. Increased endoglin enhances production of the peptide angiogenin II that increases vasoconstriction of blood vessels and promotes increased blood pressure and leads to decreased blood flow to specific sites.

Specific factors that lead to increased release of anti-angiogenic factors by the placenta have not been defined. However, lack of sufficient blood flow to the placenta may play a role. Lack of sufficient blood flow to the placenta may be due to abnormalities in the processing of the uterine arteries that normally occurs early in pregnancy. Modern ultrasound Doppler studies have revealed decreased bloodflow to the placenta in cases of pre-eclampsia. Other pre-eclampsia predisposing factors include genetic susceptibility, and immunologic factors play roles.

There are currently no specific treatments available for pre-eclampsia. Patients are encouraged to reduce salt intake and to ensure that their calcium intake is adequate. The monitoring of blood pressure and proteinuria during pregnancy is important. In cases where manifestations of pre-eclampsia are escalating, labor must be induced in adequate health care facilities. Specific treatment measures are instituted if eclamptic seizures commence. These treatments include medication to reduce brain swelling and anti-convulsants.

Uterine Rupture

Berhe and Wall (2014) reviewed causes of rupture of the uterus associated with pregnancy. They noted that uterine rupture remains a major obstetric problem in resource-poor countries. There it occurs most frequently in women who have had multiple pregnancies, with lack of antenatal care and poor access to trained birth attendants. In higher resource countries it occurs more often in women who have had previous cesarean section.

Genetic disorders that increase the risk of uterine rupture and pregnancy associated complications:

Several rare genetic disorders causing defects in connective tissue are associated with increased risks for specific pregnancy-associated complications. These disorders include Marfan syndrome, Loeys–Dietz syndrome, and the vascular type of Ehlers–Danlos syndrome. Individuals with Marfan syndrome are tall, slender and have long fingers and toes and an arm span that exceeds their height. In Marfan syndrome, defects in a specific protein (fibrillin) causes connective tissue in various part of the body to have reduced capacity to sustain stress (Dietz, 1992). This leads to weakness in vessel walls, particularly in large vessels such as the aorta. Loeys–Dietz syndrome is also associated with weakened collagen due to defects in at least four different genes that encode products in a signaling pathway that impacts connective tissue. Marfan syndrome and Loeys–Dietz syndrome may lead to aortic rupture or dissection during pregnancy and labor. Loeys–Dietz syndrome has also been associated with uterine rupture (MacCarrick, 2014).

There are six major types of Ehlers–Danlos syndrome. This syndrome results from defects in specific forms of collagen. It may also arise due to defects in proteins that bind to and modify collagen and promote its stability. Murray et al. (2014) reported that, in a survey of families with the vascular type of Ehlers–Danlos syndrome, pregnancy-related deaths occurred in 30 of 565 deliveries. In addition, there were non-lethal delivery related complications. These complications included uterine rupture, aorta or other arterial rupture, severe lacerations on vaginal delivery and failure of cesarean section incision to heal. The vascular form of Ehlers–Danlos syndrome is due to defects in the COL3A form of collagen.

Maternal Morbidity and Mortality during Labor and Delivery and in the Post-partum Period

The Executive Summary of the Lancet Maternal Survival Series (2006) reported that the leading causes of maternal death during labor and delivery and in the immediate post-partum period were severe bleeding, hypertensive disease and infection.

Uterine rupture is a very uncommon condition in developed countries, and when it does occur in those countries it usually occurs in women who have had previous deliveries by Caesarean section. However, uterine rupture is still a major cause of maternal mortality and morbidity in countries with poor resources. Mishra *et al.* (2006) reported that, in a referral hospital in Dharan, Nepal, 52 women died of uterine rupture in a four-year period. They reported that most of these women had not had prenatal care and they had commenced labor in the absence of a skilled birth attendant. They were only transferred to the hospital after prolonged labor. The maternal death rate and the fetal/infant death rate was 94.2%. Mishra *et al.* noted that many maternal deaths occurred in the rural areas of Nepal and were not reported in official statistics.

Hardee *et al.* (2012) reported that, in developing countries, reports revealed that 350,000 women died annually from pregnancy-related causes. Hardee *et al.* emphasized that maternal morbidity also remained an important problem. Significant maternal morbidity problems included the presence of fistulae between the vagina and bladder or vagina and rectum that developed as the result of obstructed labor. Estimates of the numbers of cases of such fistulae ranged between 654,000 and 2 million; 262,000 cases occurred in sub-Saharan Africa. Anemia, particularly iron deficiency anemia, was estimated to occur in 42% of pregnant woman. Maternal mental health issues were also reported to constitute significant problems.

Measures to Reduce Maternal Mortality and Morbidity

Measures to reduce maternal mortality and morbidity were included in the Millennium Development Goals (MDG) proposed by the United Nations. The target for MDG5A was to reduce maternal mortality ratio by three quarters between 1990 and 2015.

In May 2015, the WHO reported that some countries in Asia and North Africa had more than halved their maternal mortality rates. In sub-Saharan Africa, the maternal death rate was still 1 in 38. In the developed world, the maternal mortality rate is 1 in 3,700.

The 2015 WHO report noted that 10% of all women in the world did not have access to or did not use effective contraception. The Global strategy for Women's and Children's Health aimed to prevent 33 million unwanted pregnancies between 2011 and 2015. This reduction would save lives of women who would be at risk of dying during pregnancy, in childbirth or as a result of unsafe abortion.

Other Millennium Development goals that, if achieved, would greatly benefit maternal survival include MDGs 1, 3, 4 and 6. These goals are as described below.

MDG 1: Eradicate extreme poverty and hunger.

MDG 3: Promote gender equality and empower women. Women's low status, especially lack of education, contributes to and is exacerbated by high rates of maternal mortality.

MDG 4: Reduce child mortality. Good quality care for pregnant women and mothers will reduce the huge burden of neonatal deaths and improved maternal survival will enhance the survival and well-being of young children.

MDG5a Reduce by three quarters, between 1990 and 2015, the maternal mortality ratio.

MDG5b Achieve, by 2015, universal access to reproductive health.

MDG 6: Combat HIV/AIDS, Malaria and other diseases; prevent mother to child transmission of HIV and other sexually transmitted diseases.

Data have been gathered to determine evidence of progress toward achieving these MDG goals. In some areas, post 2015-era strategies have been formulated.

In 2014, Lawn et al. wrote: "The Millennium Development goals have driven global priorities in countries. Donor funding for reproductive maternal and child health has doubled". The Lawn et al. report noted, however, that there were still 2.9 million infant deaths during the first 28 days after birth; 800,000 neonatal deaths occurred among babies born small for gestational age. The five countries with the highest burdens of neonatal deaths were reported to be India, Nigeria, Pakistan, China and the Democratic Republic of Congo. Neonatal death rates are also high in Lesotho and Angola. It is important to note, however, that stillbirths and neonatal death rates are often inaccurately reported in many countries.

The leading causes of neonatal deaths included severe infection, intra-partum or preterm birth complications. Intra-partum conditions included asphyxia.

6 Newborn Infants: Prematurity and Other Problems

In January 1966, I started work as a temporary house officer in the Department of Pediatrics in Hospitals affiliated with Glasgow University, Scotland. My first assignment was at the Queen Mother's Maternity Hospital. Our main duties as house officers included care of infants in a unit specially dedicated to the care of premature infants and newborns at risk due to problems that were detected at birth or early after birth.

Dr. Margaret Kerr served as the senior physician in charge of that special unit. She was deeply devoted to the care of premature and fragile infants. Under her supervision and together with the skilled nurses, we house officers worked to try to address the main problems in these infants. Problems included respiratory difficulties, feeding difficulties and maintenance of normal body temperature. We monitored the infants to be sure they did not become cyanotic due to diminished respiratory function. In addition, we monitored them for jaundice and for measured bilirubin levels. Bilirubin is derived from red cell breakdown. It is usually processed in the liver and then excreted primarily in the gut and also in the urine. In immature infants, the liver may not be able to adequately process the bilirubin derived from red cell breakdown. High levels of unprocessed bilirubin (unconjugated bilirubin) can damage the brain. Problems with increased levels of unconjugated bilirubin were particularly common in infants where there were maternal-fetal blood group incompatibilities present. These incompatibilities led to increased breakdown of blood cells in fetuses and newborn infants. In Scotland at that time, fetal maternal blood incompatibility problems mainly arose in mothers who were negative for the Rhesus (Rh) blood group and had infants who were positive for Rh blood group.

If the bilirubin level rose above 20, infants needed an exchange blood transfusion to rid their systems of the damaging breakdown product. Exchange transfusion was a delicate procedure and it was usually carried out by the head physician. I remember how skillful Dr. Margaret Kerr was at catheterizing the small blood vessels that could be accessed in the remnant of the umbilical cord. She would sit for hours slowly drawing out a small quantity of blood from one umbilical vessel and then slowly injecting the same quantity of blood group matched donor blood into a second umbilical vessel. The infant was kept warm and well oxygenated and carefully monitored for ill effects.

The newborn special care unit was located on the top floor of the Queen Mother's hospital and it had spacious windows with a view of the busy docks and shipyards of Glasgow. I still remember the strange sensations and emotions I felt when, after concentrating for hours on the fragile infant to monitor heart rate, temperature and breathing without the use of modern electronic equipment, I would move away from the crib and look out the windows to see the giant works of man: large ships, cranes and engines.

It was interesting later to refresh my memory of hemolytic disease of the newborn. In 1932, Louis Diamond made the connection between unusual levels of red cell breakdown in infants, referred to as hemolytic disease of the newborn, the rise in levels of unconjugated bilirubin (the less soluble form of bilirubin), and deposition of this in the brain. This deposition could lead to brain damage, spasticity, movement disorders and delayed development. In 1941, Levine first discovered that hemolysis occurred when the Rh negative mother who had been immunized to Rh positive cells during a previous pregnancy, and who carried a Rh positive fetus in a subsequent pregnancy. In a mother who carried high concentrations of anti-Rh antibodies, hemolysis could start occurring in the second fetus. Great advances came when pregnant women were tested for Rh blood group status in pregnancy, and with the development of Rh antiserum Rhogam (Freda et al., 1964).

Ideally, women who are Rh negative are given an antiserum Rhogam after delivery in their first pregnancy to destroy any remaining fetal blood cells that had landed in the maternal circulation during the birth process. The antibodies present in Rhogam are short lived in the maternal circulation. They do, however, serve to destroy the remaining fetal cells before they elicit an immune response. Rhogam was first used in 1968. Rhogam injection immediately after delivery of an infant or immediately after a miscarriage has greatly reduced the incidence of hemolytic disease of the newborn (Bowman, 2006).

The Rh blood group seemed straightforward initially. Individuals were Rh positive if they carried one gene or two genes (one on each member of the chromosome 1 pair) that produced a specific protein, the Rh antigen. Molecular genetic studies revealed that the Rh system is more complicated. Colin (in 1991) determined that there are two linked genes that produce Rh antigens. In Rh positive individuals there is an RHD gene which encodes the RhD protein, and a second gene that encodes both the RhC and RhE antigens on a single polypeptide. In Caucasians who are RhD antigen negative, the RHD gene is deleted. In RhD positive individuals there is at least one RHD gene with 10 coding segments (exons) (Fasano, 2016).

Rh negative individuals also occur in African populations. In the majority of African Rh negative individuals there is a pseudo RHD gene. The RHD pseudogene has structural changes including duplication of specific exons, and in some individuals the RHD pseudogene is a hybrid and has exons from RHD fused to exons from RHCE. Neither of these RHD pseudogenes produces Rh antigens.

Rh testing is usually done on blood cells and depends on Rh antigens present on these cells. Fasano reported new approaches to the Rh problems, including the paternal Rh status in Rh negative women who do not have anti-Rh antibodies. It is now also possible to determine the fetal blood type through genotyping, by sampling of fetal DNA that is now known to be present in maternal blood (Fasano, 2016).

It is important to note that hemolytic disease of the newborn may rarely be due to maternal-fetal incompatibilities of other blood group antigens. It is also important to emphasize that neonatal jaundice (hyperbilirubinemia) may be related to impaired, or immature, liver function.

Prematurity and Causes

Lawn *et al.* (2014) reported evidence that girls who became pregnant before 18 years of age are at higher risk for maternal morbidity and mortality. In addition, risks are higher in these cases for stillbirths, preterm birth, neonatal deaths and for delivery of infants small for gestational age. They note that social norms such as child marriage and genital mutilation are also associated with adverse pregnancy outcomes. There is also evidence that communities with the highest fertility rates and birth rates and that lack access to family planning have the highest rates of neonatal deaths.

Preterm Birth in Developed Countries

Blencowe et al. (2013) classified preterm births into two broad subtypes:

1. Spontaneous preterm birth due to premature onset of uterine contractions, premature rupture of membranes.
2. Provider-initiated preterm birth, induction of labor or elective cesarean section birth before 37 weeks of gestation are completed, for maternal or for fetal indications or other non-medical reasons.

Spontaneous Preterm Birth

Blencowe et al. reported that in more than 50% of cases the causes of preterm birth remained unidentified. Maternal history of a prior preterm birth is a strong risk factor. Other specific risk factors include very young maternal age or advanced maternal age. Pregnancies with multiple fetuses are also at increased risk for preterm birth. Infections, excessive physical work and prolonged standing likely also act as risk factors.

The authors noted an increase in the number of twin and triplet pregnancies in recent years. In England, Wales and France this was most likely due to increased use of in vitro fertilization and implantation of multiple embryos.

Blencowe et al. noted that unintended preterm birth occurred in some cases of provider-initiated delivery when gestational age was incorrectly accessed. The current best estimate of gestational age is based on an algorithm that includes date of last menstrual period and ultrasound measurements of fetal growth.

Medically indicated reasons for provider-initiated preterm birth include pre-eclampsia, abnormal placental position or function and fetal growth restriction. Other maternal health conditions associated with preterm birth include cardiac conditions and diabetes. In some women cervical incompetence leads to preterm birth.

In 2013, Blencowe *et al.* reported that world-wide preterm births occurred in 14.9 million babies and overall preterm births occurred in 11.1% of pregnancies. The highest rates of preterm births occurred in South Asia and sub-Saharan Africa, where premature births occurred in 13.4% of pregnancies. In high-income countries, 1.2 million preterm births occurred and 42% of these were in the USA. They noted that preterm birth rates, particularly rates of birth between 32 and 37 weeks, increased in Europe, in the Americas and in Australasia between 1990 and 2010.

Preterm Births in the USA

In an Institute of Medicine report from 2007, Behrman *et al.* reported that in the USA the preterm birthrate was highest in African American women, and it occurred in 17.8% of their pregnancies. The preterm birthrate for white American women was 11.5%, and it was slightly lower in Asian American women and Pacific Islanders.

Russell *et al.* (2006) reported that in the USA the average hospital costs in cases of preterm births and low birthweight infants was $15,000, while hospital costs for term infant births and hospital admissions for approximately 2 days was $600. For extremely preterm infants at less than 28 weeks' gestation and with birthweights less than 1000 g, hospital costs averaged $65,600.

Survival Rates of Preterm Infants

Lawn *et al.* (2013) reported that in low income countries approximately half of all babies born at 32 weeks' or less gestation died. Complications associated with preterm births potentially involved the respiratory, gastro-intestinal and central nervous systems. Their report emphasized that the greatest mortality rate was in infants born at the earliest gestational age.

The Institute of Medicine report noted that there is evidence that preterm birth infants who survive the neonatal period and the first few weeks may have long-term problems that continue beyond infancy. These include cognitive and behavioral problems, vision and hearing problems and growth defects. School-age children with a history of preterm birth also frequently require additional services. There is evidence that infants born near to term experience more difficulties than infants born at term.

7 Neural Tube Defects

My own encounters with neural tube defects occurred in two locations very distant from each other. As a young physician employed as a house officer at the Queen Mother's hospital in Glasgow, Scotland, ward round duties for a short time included a visit to a single infant in a separate room located distant from the regular nurseries. This infant was born with anencephaly, a form of neural tube defect where the top of the skull and brain had not developed properly. Anencephaly frequently leads to stillbirth; anencephalic infants born alive die within a few days or weeks. I was deeply moved by the attention the nurses gave to this infant in the isolated room. One nurse told me that they had been instructed not to feed the anencephalic infant. However, the infant made soft sounds and when offered bottle feed it seems the infant sucked for brief periods. The parents of this infant were deeply distressed as they waited for the inevitable death of their child.

Many years later, while working as a genetics physician in California, I encountered an infant with anencephaly who lived for about one week after his birth. This infant was in a crib in a nursery along with other infants. The nurses had found a brightly colored knitted baby's cap to cover the head above the eyes and face.

As a member of the Genetics division in the early 1980s I participated as a member of the team of physicians who provided services to patients and families in the Spina Bifida clinic. The team also included neurologists, neurosurgeons, urologists, nurses and social workers. As geneticists our role was to record family histories, pregnancy and birth histories and to examine patients for the possible presence of congenital malformations not directly related to spina bifida.

The team in the spina bifida clinic worked well together. Neurosurgeons and orthopedic surgeons provided valuable services to patients who required surgeries to address the spinal defects. Neurosurgeons were often called upon to install shunts for spina bifida patients who had excessive accumulation of cerebrospinal fluid in the brain (hydrocephalus), that occurred secondarily to the neural tube defect. In some cases, orthopedists could recommend procedures and bracing to partially manage lower limb defects and paralysis. The urologists provided important services in dealing with bladder-related problems that arose due to impaired nerve supply to the bladder. The skilled nurses and social workers coordinated the efforts of the whole team and made sure that families had access to services and provisions available to them through the state program, The California Children's services.

Over the years, the numbers of infants and children needing service in Spina Bifida clinics declined; the discoveries that led to declining of these needs are described below.

Reducing the risk of neural tube defects through adequate folate intake:

Chris Schorah (2011) traced the history of efforts to reduce the incidence of neural tube defects. He wrote: "the 'apparent' prevention of neural tube defects (NTDs) with periconceptual vitamin supplements was to become 'actual' prevention. But it was a long day's journey into light".

In 1965, Hibbard and Smithells published an article in the Lancet that drew attention to the relationship of defects in embryonic development and abnormal folate metabolism. In 1976, Smithells *et al.* published results of studies on levels of serum folate, red cell folate, vitamin C, vitamin A and riboflavin levels in 900 pregnant women and they monitored fetuses and infants at birth. Their study revealed that in mothers who gave birth to infants with neural tube defects, the red cell folate levels during the first trimester of pregnancy were significantly lower than the levels in women who gave birth to normal infants. Smithells *et al.* concluded that these findings indicated that vitamin supplements that contained folate significantly reduced the incidence of neural tube defects. Their conclusions met with vehement opposition.

In 1980, Smithells *et al.* published results of a study in which women that had previously given birth to a child with neural tube defects were offered a trial of periconceptual multivitamin supplements that included folic acid for 28 days prior to conception and continuing into the first months of pregnancy. The control group included women who refused to take the periconceptual vitamins. Results of their study revealed that in the group of 176 women who chose supplements only one infant was born with neural tube defect. In the control group of 160 women who refused supplementation, 13 cases with neural tube defects occurred.

In 1981, the British Medical Research Council proposed a double blind randomized trial that included one group of women given vitamin supplementation that included folic acid in the periconceptual and early pregnancy period and another group not given supplementation. Results of this trial were not reported until 1992.

Fortunately, in 1984 Seller and Nevin reported in the medical literature results of supplementation studies in reducing the rate of recurrent neural tube defects in South-East England and Ireland.

The final report of the MRC double blind study (MRC Vitamin Study Research Group (1991)) indicated that more than 70% of cases of neural tube defects could be prevented by intake of 400 micrograms of folate per day during the periconceptual period and early pregnancy.

In 1992, the Public Health Service in the USA (https://www.uspre-ventiveservicestaskforce.org/) recommended that women capable of becoming pregnant consume 400 micrograms of folic acid per day. In 1998, the government of the USA mandated fortification of cereal grain products with folic acid.

The Brownsville Texas cluster of Neural Tube defects:
In 1991, the Texas state health department was contacted by a physician who reported that within a 36-hour period three anencephalic infants were born in a single hospital in Brownsville, Texas. This report was followed by a surveillance of the county in which Brownsville was located, and the prevalence of neural tube defects was found to be 29 infants in 10,000 births. This was the highest recorded prevalence of neural tube defects in the USA since the 1970s; a six-year case control study was initiated. In 2012, Suarez et al. reviewed comprehensive results of this study, that investigated nutrient and micronutrient intake, maternal health status, biochemical markers and environmental factors. In the Mexican–American population in Brownsville, corn tortillas were a staple food.

Results of the study confirmed that increased folate intake had a protective effect against neural tube defects. The study also noted that in mothers' low serum vitamin B12 levels, high serum homocysteine levels and maternal obesity contributed to neural tube defect risk. Other neural tube risk factors that emerged from this study included food contamination with fumonisin mold and high nitrate and nitrite levels in water.

Suarez *et al.* concluded that neural tube defects were multifactorial in etiology and that deficiency of folic acid in the diet increased vulnerability to neural tube defects.

A 2015 report from the USA Center for Disease Control (CDC) (www. cdc.gov/NCBDDD/folicacid/data.html) noted that there was a significant decline in the incidence of neural tube defects in all population groups in the years following folic acid fortification of grain cereals. In addition, studies on blood folate levels also revealed significant declines in evidence of folate deficiency following fortification. However, the prevalence of neural tube defects continued to be higher in the Hispanic population than in other USA population groups.

Fumonisins (produced by *Fusarium* fungus) are known to produce an enzyme that inhibits the synthesis of sphingolipids, that are key components of cell membranes and particularly of myelin in the central and peripheral nervous systems (Marasas *et al.*, 2004). It turns out that fumonisin exposure possibly also play a role in the etiology of neural tube defects.

World-wide Studies on Neural Tube Defects

Blencowe *et al.* (2010) reported that the burden of Neural Tube Defects in low income countries continued to be high. They estimated that folic acid fortification could prevent 13% of deaths attributed to congenital malformations.

Pathogenesis of Neural Tube Defects

Neural tube defects arise due to defects in the processes of folding and fusion of the neural plate that forms in early embryogenesis. The process of fusing of the edges of the neural plate occurs at several sites in the brain region and along the spine. Failure of appropriate fusion in the head region leads to anencephaly. Failure of fusion at sites in the spinal regions leads to spina bifida (Greene and Copp, 2014).

In spina bifida the vertebral column does not adequately cover the underlying neural tissue. The neural tissue that protrudes through the spinal column may be covered by meningeal membranes. The presence of the neural tube defect may impact the flow of cerebrospinal fluid and be associated with increased cerebro-spinal fluid in the brain (hydrocephalus). In some cases, the neural tissue may be covered by malformed vertebrae and skin, leading to closed neural tube defects.

Measurable Markers of Neural Tube Defects during Pregnancy

In 1972, Brock and Sutcliffe reported that analysis of a specific protein in amniotic fluid, alpha-fetoprotein, revealed that increased levels of this protein occurred in the presence of fetuses with open neural tube defect. Subsequently, maternal serum levels of the fetal protein alpha-fetoprotein were also shown to be elevated in pregnancies with fetuses with open neural tube defects (Brock *et al.*, 1973). However, raised levels of alpha-fetoprotein also occur in association with a number of other birth defects.

8 Thyroid Hormone Deficiency in Infants and Children

My most memorable experience of thyroid hormone deficiency occurred when I was a house officer at the Yorkhill Children's Hospital in Glasgow. Three siblings were admitted to the hospital at the same time. The eldest, a girl of 12 years of age, manifested symptoms of severe thyroid hormone deficiency: growth retardation, intellectual impairments, and thickening of the tissues of the face and neck. These features had in previous decades been referred to as manifestations of cretinism. The second sibling, a girl of nine years of age, had evidence of growth retardation and some evidence of developmental delay. The youngest sibling, a boy of five years of age, had growth delay. On laboratory testing, all three children were found to have thyroid hormone deficiency. They were children of a couple who travelled around in a caravan and who had no fixed address. The children did not have regular medical care and they did not attend school. The three siblings were devoted to each other. Although they each had separate beds in the hospital ward, we would regularly find them huddled together in one bed if we entered the ward late at night or early in the morning. The children were thought to have a defect in a biochemical process that leads to iodination of thyroid hormone in the thyroid gland. Their deficiency of active thyroid hormone could be readily compensated for with treatment using thyroid hormone pills. It was also particularly important to gain the parents' confidence in order to persuade them to work with us, and subsequently with district nurses and facilities where they located to, in order to ensure ongoing care of the children and continued access to the required medication.

Some years later, starting in 1981, my duties as a physician in the department of Pediatrics at the University of California, Irvine included services in the California Newborn Screening Program. In this program, newborns are screened for conditions that if present can be readily treated early in infancy, thereby preventing handicaps with life-long consequences. Specific genetic conditions were screened for and I will describe these in a later chapter. Newborn heel stick blood samples were also screened to detect thyroid hormone deficiency. Neonatal screening for hypothyroidism was first initiated in Canada in 1972 and results were reported by Dussault et al. (1975). Failure to diagnose thyroid hormone deficiency very early in life can cause infants and children to suffer impaired neurological and physical development.

In our program, following notification from the California Newborn Screening Program that an infant born in our county, Orange County, had been found to have an abnormal result we contacted the child's physician. If the physician could not be reached we contacted the family directly so that the child could be referred to an endocrinologist for assessment and therapy.

I noted with interest a 2013 report by a physician from Turkey, Atilla Buyukgebiz who wrote:

"Newborn screening for congenital hypothyroidism is one of the major achievements of preventive medicine. Although since 1972 the problem of congenital hypothyroidism has been resolved in developed countries the same cannot be said of developing countries that still have no newborn screening programs for congenital hypothyroidism".

Historical Discoveries Related to Hypothyroidism

The history of hypothyroidism, in past decades referred to as cretinism with goiter, is fascinating. Merke compiled in 1960 a richly illustrated volume entitled: "History and Iconography of Endemic Goiter and Cretinism". He collected photos of statue images and paintings, dating from the medieval period on, of people with the enlarged neck swelling referred to as goiters. Goiters were particularly common in the mountainous regions of Europe: in Switzerland, Burgundy, Southern Tyrol, the Lombardy region of Italy and in regions close to the Pyrenees mountains on the border between France and Spain.

In 1825, a Frenchman J. Boussingault documented that he had followed up on information he obtained from people in Columbia, South America, that ash from seaweed and sponges was beneficial in treating a goitrous disorder that was common in people living in mountainous regions. Boussingault analyzed the material from seaweed and sponges and reported that it was high in iodine and that it cured goiters. Cesar Lombroso promoted the use of iodine for the treatment of goiter in Switzerland in 1873.

In 1895, Bauman reported that a high concentration of iodine occurred in thyroid glands. Raw or lightly cooked sheep thyroid was used in treatment of cretinism in the 1890s. Cretinism occurred sporadically in Britain. Ireland wrote in 1898 of success in treatment with developmental delay and features of cretinism:

"Results of such treatment are so rapid and striking that they resemble the transformation in a fairy tale rather than the slow gains of the healing art against chronic disease".

He noted further, however:

"It has been a disappointment to our warm hopes that under thyroid treatment the mental improvement has not kept pace with bodily growth though almost all patients have shown a quickening of intelligence. Naturally the improvement has been greater the earlier the age at which they were treated".

Isolation of the hormone thyroxin, (tetraiodothyronine) from the thyroid was reported by Kendall in 1915. Harrington and Berger (1927) reported on the chemical structures of the different forms of thyroxin, T3 and T4, in 1925.

Early experiments on tadpoles carried out independently by Allen (1916) and Smith (1916) revealed that the pituitary gland in the brain produced a substance that stimulated the thyroid gland and was necessary for the metamorphosis of tadpole into frog. However, isolation of the pituitary-derived factor that stimulated the thyroid gland was only achieved in the 1950s. In reviewing the history of its discovery, Magner (2014) noted that isolation of thyroid stimulating hormone (TSH) required application of specific protein separation technology, namely ion exchange chromatography. The TSH protein was found to be composed of alpha and beta subunits.

The brain regions that influence production of thyroid stimulating hormone include the hypothalamus and the pituitary. Although most cases of congenital hypothyroidism are due to defects in development or functioning of the thyroid gland, there are rare cases that are due to impaired function of the pituitary, or impaired functioning of the hypothalamic–pituitary axis. These cases are referred to as cases of Central Hypothyroidism. Unfortunately, such cases are missed in certain newborn screening programs that screen only for the raised levels of thyroid stimulating hormone (TSH) that occur in the more common forms of hypothyroidism that are due to developmental defects of the thyroid gland or defects in function of the thyroid. In cases of central hypothyroidism, the TSH levels are clearly not elevated.

In the Netherlands, the incidence of Central Hypothyroidism was reported as 1 in 16,000 newborns. The incidence of hypothyroidism due to defective formation or function of the thyroid gland is reported as ranging between 1 in 1,600 newborns and 1 in 3,000 newborns. Raised levels of TSH and transient hypothyroidism occur in premature infants (Garcia et al., 2014),

Hypothalamic–pituitary Axis and Thyroid Function

The paraventricular nucleus of the anterior hypothalamus produces a specific hormone, thyroid releasing hormone (TRH). This hormone passes to the pituitary gland where it binds to a specific receptor, the thyroid releasing hormone receptor (TRHR), that is located on specific cells known as thyrotropes. On binding of TRH to the receptor, the thyrotrope cells are activated and they produce thyroid stimulating hormone (TSH).

Defects in production of thyroid stimulating hormone leading to central hypothyroidism may result from defects in development of the pituitary. In these cases, there may also be defects in production of other pituitary hormones. Abnormalities in pituitary development are, in some cases, due to mutations in specific transcription factors or specific signaling molecules involved in pituitary development.

Deficiency of thyroid stimulating hormone and central hypothyroidism may also result from mutations in genes that encode the thyroid hormone releasing factor or genes that encode the receptor for thyroid hormone releasing factor (Garcia et al., 2014).

Defects in synthesis of thyroid hormone by the thyroid gland:

Congenital hypothyroidism may be due to complete or partial absence of the thyroid gland. In most cases, congenital hypothyroidism is sporadic, however inherited forms of hypothyroidism occur. Genetic mutations may lead to defects in proteins or enzymes involved in the synthesis of active thyroid hormones. This synthesis requires initial coupling of the thyroid stimulating hormone (TSH) to a TSH binding receptor (TSHR) on thyroid gland cells and synthesis of thyroglobulin by the thyroid cells. Other critical processes involved in the synthesis of active thyroid hormone include the transport of iodine into the thyroid with specific transporters, modification of iodine and coupling of modified iodine to tyrosine residues present in thyroglobulin (Szinnai, 2014).

Modification of iodine and its coupling to tyrosine are dependent on the presence of hydrogen peroxide in the thyroid gland cells and on the activity of a specific enzyme, thyroid peroxidase (TPO). Hydrogen peroxide generation in the thyroid is dependent on the presence of specific enzymes referred to as dual oxidase.

Deficiency of iodine or defects in any one of the genes that encode the products required for synthesis of active thyroid hormone can lead to hypothyroidism. Goiter, enlargement of the thyroid gland, occurs in situations where the levels of circulating hormone are low and thyroid stimulating hormone is secreted by the pituitary in efforts to increase thyroid hormone levels.

Iodine Deficiency in Recent Decades

Consistent efforts have been made by the WHO, by non-profit organizations such as UNICEF and by governmental public health agencies to increase iodine intake though iodization of salt.

In 1991, the BBC, London presented a program entitled "The Rain Plague". The presenters related how, in a specific community in Bangladesh, cretinism occurred in children following a decision by the village elders to stop purchasing iodized salt because it was costlier than non-iodized salt.

In 2008, de Benoist et al. published data on global iodine deficiency. They reported that mild to moderate iodine deficiency was present in North-East Asia, in the Soviet Union, in some countries of Eastern Europe and in regions of Africa.

A WHO report on micronutrient deficiencies indicated that the number of countries where iodine deficiency is a public health problem has halved in recent decades. However, iodine deficiency was still present in 54 countries and continued efforts are required in those countries to strengthen salt iodization programs.

References

Allen BM. (1916). Extirpation of the hypophysis and thyroid glands of Rana pipiens. *Anat Rec* **11**:486.

Bauman E. (1895). Uber das normale vorkommen van Jod im Thierkorper. *Z Physiol Chem* **21** (319).

BBC (1991). The rain plague, www.worldcat.org/title/rain-plague/oclc/51663689.

Behrman RE, Butler AS. eds. (2007). *Preterm Birth: Causes, Consequences, and Prevention.* Washington (DC): National Academies Press (US).

Berhe Y, Wall LL. (2014). Uterine rupture in resource-poor countries. *Obstet Gynecol Surv* **69(11):**695–707. doi: 10.1097/OGX.0000000000000123. PMID:25409161.

Blencowe H, Cousens S, Chou D, *et al.* (2013). Born too soon: the global epidemiology of 15 million preterm births. *Reprod Health* **10** Suppl 1:S2. doi: 10.1186/1742-4755-10-S1-S2. PMID:24625129.

Blencowe H, Cousens S, Modell B, Lawn J. (2010). Folic acid to reduce neonatal mortality from neural tube disorders. *Int J Epidemiol* **39** Suppl 1:i110–21. doi: 10.1093/ije/dyq028. PMID:20348114.

Boussingault JB. (1825). Goitre prophylaxis. *Annales de chimie et de physique* **40**.

Bowman J. (2006). Rh-immunoglobulin: Rh prophylaxis. *Best Pract Res Clin Haematol* **19(1):**27–34. PMID:16377539.

Brock DJ, Sutcliffe RG. (1972). Alpha-fetoprotein in the antenatal diagnosis of anencephaly and spina bifida. *Lancet* **Jul 29;2(7770):**197–9. PMID:4114207.

Brock DJ, Bolton AE, Monaghan JM. (1973). Prenatal diagnosis of anencephaly through maternal serum-alphafetoprotein measurement. *Lancet* **Oct 27;2(7835):**923–4. PMID:4126556.

Büyükgebiz A. (2013). Newborn screening for congenital hypothyroidism. *J Clin Res Pediatr Endocrinol* **5 Suppl 1:**8–12. doi: 10.4274/jcrpe.845. PMID:23154158.

Colin Y, Chérif-Zahar B, Le Van Kim C, *et al.* (1991). Genetic basis of the RhD-positive and RhD-negative blood group polymorphism as determined by Southern analysis. *Blood* **Nov 15;78(10):**2747–52. PMID:1824267.

de Benoist B, McLean E, Andersson M, Rogers L. (2008). Iodine deficiency in 2007: global progress since 2003. *Food Nutr Bull* **Sep;29(3):**195–202. PMID:18947032.

Diamond LK, KD Blackfan, JM Baty (1932). Erythroblastosis fetalis and its association with universal edema of the fetus, icterus gravis neonatorum and anemia of the newborn. *The Journal of Pediatrics* **1(3):**269–309.

Dietz HC. (1992). Molecular biology of Marfan syndrome. *J Vasc Surg* **15(5):**927–8.

Duley L. (2009). The global impact of pre-eclampsia and eclampsia. *Semin Perinatol* **33(3):**130–7. doi: 10.1053/j.semperi.2009.02.010. PMID:19464502.

Executive Summary of The Lancet Maternal Survival Series http://www.familycareintl.org/UserFiles/File/MaternalSurvExecSum%20FINAL.pdf

Fasano RM. (2016). Hemolytic disease of the fetus and newborn in the molecular era. *Semin Fetal Neonatal Med* **21(1)**:28–34. doi: 10.1016/j.siny.2015.10.006. PMID:26589360.

Freda VJ, Gorman JG, Pollack W. (1964). Successful prevention of experimental Rh sensitization in man with an anti-Rh gamma 2-globulin antibody preparation: a preliminary report. *Transfusion* **4**:26.

Dussault JH, Coulombe P, Laberge C, *et al*. (1975). Preliminary report on a mass screening program for neonatal hypothyroidism. *J Pediatr* **86(5)**:670–4. PMID:1133648.

García M, Fernández A, Moreno JC. (2014). Central hypothyroidism in children. *Endocr Dev* **26**:79–107. doi: 10.1159/000363157. PMID:25231446.

Greene ND, Copp AJ. (2014). Neural tube defects. *Annu Rev Neurosci* **37**:221–42. doi: 10.1146/annurev-neuro-062012-170354. PMID:25032496.

Hardee K, Gay J, Blanc AK. (2012). Maternal morbidity: neglected dimension of safe motherhood in the developing world. *Glob Public Health* **7(6)**:603–17. doi: 10.1080/17441692.2012.668919.

Harington CR, Barger G. (1927). Chemistry of Thyroxine Constitution and Synthesis of Thyroxine. *Biochem J* **21(1)**:169–183. PMCID: PMC1251886.

Hibbard ED, Smithells RW. (1965). Folic acid metabolism and human embryopathy. *Lancet* **285(7398)**:1254. doi:10.1016/S0140-6736(65)91895-7.

Ireland WW. (1898). *Mental affections of Children*. London: J and A Churchill, p243 and p245.

Kendall E. (1915). The isolation in crystalline form of the compound containing iodine, which occurs in the thyroid. Its chemical nature and physiologic activity. *JAMA* **64**:2042–3.

Lawn JE, Blencowe H, Oza S *et al*. (2014). (Lancet Every Newborn Study Group) Every Newborn: progress, priorities, and potential beyond survival. *Lancet* **384(9938)**:189–205. doi: 10.1016/S0140-6736(14)60496-7. Erratum in: Lancet. 2014 Jul 12;384(9938):132. PMID:24853593.

Levine P, Vogel P, Katzin EM, Burnham L. (1941). Pathogenesis of erythroblastosis fetalis: statistical evidence. *Science* **94(2442)**:371–372.

Lombroso C. (1873). Sulla microcephalia e sul cretinismo. Rivista Clinica di Bologua fasc. 7 July.

MacCarrick G, Black JH 3rd, Bowdin S, *et al*. (2014). Loeys-Dietz syndrome: a primer for diagnosis and management. *Genet Med* **16(8)**:576–87. doi: 10.1038/gim.2014.11. PMID:24577266.

Magner J. (2014). Historical note: many steps led to the 'discovery' of thyroid-stimulating hormone. *Eur Thyroid J* **3(2)**:95–100. doi: 10.1159/000360534. PMID:25114872.

Marasas WF, Riley RT, Hendricks KA, *et al*. (2004). Fumonisins disrupt sphingo-lipid metabolism, folate transport, and neural tube development in embryo culture and in vivo: a potential risk factor for human neural tube defects among populations consuming fumonisin-contaminated maize. *J Nutr* **134(4):**711–6. PMID:15051815.

MDG 5: Improve maternal health. http://www.who.int/topics/millennium_development_goals/maternal_health/en/

Merke F. (1960). The history of endemic goitre and cretinism in the thirteenth to fifteenth centuries. *Proc R Soc Med* **53(12):**995–1002. PMID:13769623.

Mishra SK, Morris N, Uprety DK. (2006). Uterine rupture: preventable obstetric tragedies? *Aust N Z J Obstet Gynaecol* **46(6):**541–5. PMID:17116062.

Murray ML, Pepin M, Peterson S, Byers PH. (2014). Pregnancy-related deaths and complications in women with vascular Ehlers-Danlos syndrome. *Genet Med* **16(12):**874–80. doi: 10.1038/gim.2014.53. PMID:24922461.

Russell RB, Green NS, Steiner CA, *et al*. (2007). Cost of hospitalization for preterm and low birth weight infants in the United States. *Pediatrics* **120(1):**e1–9. PMID:17606536.

Schorah C. (2011). Commentary: from controversy and procrastination to primary prevention. *Int J Epidemiol* **40(5):**1156–8. doi: 10.1093/ije/dyr133. PMID:22039191.

Seller MJ, Nevin NC. (1984). Periconceptional vitamin supplementation and the prevention of neural tube defects in South-East England and Northern Ireland. *J Med Genet* **21(5):**325–30. PMID:6502647.

Smith PE. (1916). Experimental ablation of the hypophysis in the frog embryo. *Science* **44(1130):**280–282

Smithells RW, Sheppard S, Schorah CJ. (1976). Vitamin deficiencies and neural tube defects. *Arch Dis Child* **51(12):**944–50. PMID:1015847.

Smithells RW, Sheppard S, Schorah CJ, *et al*. (1980). Possible prevention of neural-tube defects by periconceptional vitamin supplementation. Lancet **315(8169):**647–648. PMID:6102643.

Suarez L, Felkner M, Brender JD, *et al*. (2012). Neural tube defects on the Texas-Mexico border: what we've learned in the 20 years since the Brownsville cluster. *Birth Defects Res A Clin Mol Teratol* **94(11):**882–92. doi: 10.1002/bdra.23070. PMID:22945287.

Szinnai G. (2014). Clinical genetics of congenital hypothyroidism. *Endocr Dev* **26:**60–78. doi: 10.1159/000363156. PMID:25231445.

Williams J, Mai CT, Mulinare J, *et al*. (2015). Updated Estimates of Neural Tube Defects Prevented by Mandatory Folic Acid Fortification — United States, 1995–2011. *Centers for disease control and prevention: morbidity and mortality weekly report* January 16, 2015/64(01);1–5. http://www.cdc.gov/mmwr/preview/mmwrhtml/mm6401a2.htm.

WHO: Micronutrient deficiencies. http://www.who.int/nutrition/topics/idd/en/ (Accessed on February 15th 2016).

WHO: Preterm birth. http://www.who.int/mediacentre/factsheets/fs363/en/

Young BC, Levine RJ, Kammanchi SA. (2010). Pathogenesis of preeclanpsia. *Annu Rev Pathol* **5**:173–92. doi: 10.1146/annurev-pathol-121808-102149. PMID:20078220.

PART III

Infection Related Diseases

9 Fading, Emerging and Re-emerging Infectious Diseases

I think back to my school years and to the year I worked as a house officer at the Yorkhill site of the Royal Hospital for Sick Children in Glasgow, Scotland and to memories of children with acute rheumatic fever and others with acute glomerulonephritis. These diseases occur much less frequently now, at least in Western Societies.

I remember my classmate, Thia. We were together as pupils for eight years at a convent school in a suburb of Johannesburg, South Africa. I cannot remember the exact year, it was likely 1954, when Thia became ill and was diagnosed with acute rheumatic fever and was confined to bed for almost three months. Luckily she was taken care of in her home. After her initial period of complete rest, I was able to visit her, and still later I was able to bring her books to read and news from school. We both matriculated from high school in 1957 and Thia went on to become a nurse.

I remember Anna, whom I met in the Johannesburg Children's Hospital when I was 12 years old and was admitted for acute appendicitis and surgery. In the six bed hospital ward, Anna was opposite me and we became friends. Anna had been in the hospital for many weeks. Her diagnosis was acute rheumatic fever. My hospital stay was short. After I left the hospital I wrote letters to Anna and kept in contact with her even after her hospital release. A while after that, Anna joined our family on a trip to the seaside at Umdloti beach near Durban Natal. I do not know if Anna had long term complications from rheumatic fever, such as mitral stenosis and impaired heart function.

In 1960, as a third year medical student in Pretoria, South Africa, I got to learn about the bacillus *Streptococcus* and about the important work of Griffith and Lancefield in classifying the different strains of beta-hemolytic *Streptococcus*. Lancefield determined that infections with specific strains of Group A beta-hemolytic *Streptococcus* were sometimes followed by manifestations of acute rheumatic fever. Only recently did I learn that Lancefield was a woman, Rebecca Lancefield. I tracked down her biography, including one written by Maclyn McCarty (1987), and learned of her contributions to microbiology during her long career 1918–1979.

Frederick Griffith was active in research in England between the 1920s and 1941, when he was killed in the bombing of London during the Blitz of World War II. For Frederick Griffith in England (1928) and for Rebecca Lancefield (1933) in New York, their work on *Streptococcus* was initial primarily in response to the high population frequencies of pneumonia that resulted from infection with *Streptococcus pneumoniae*, an alpha-hemolytic form of *Streptococcus*. Griffith and Lancefield used different techniques to classify streptococci, however they exchanged organisms and reagents and they reached joint conclusions.

Early work on beta-hemolytic *Streptococcus* group A revealed that infections with specific strains of that organism were followed in some cases by post-streptococcal glomerulonephritis. The glomerulonephritis associated strains were different than the rheumatic fever associated strains.

My memories of glomerulonephritis include memories of Mary, a young girl of approximately 12 years of age who was a patient at the Yorkhill branch of the Royal Hospital for Sick Children. Mary was hospitalized for several weeks. I spent time chatting with her during the few quiet intervals in my busy house officer schedule. She was fascinated by the fact that I had lived in Africa and she had many questions about wild animals. After months on the job I had a 5-day vacation and I traveled to Arran Isle off the west coast of Scotland to hike. On my return I found out that Mary's condition had deteriorated and her kidney failure was severe. Mary had been transferred from the general ward to a private room. When I called in on her she asked "Why did you leave me? I got very sick". A sense of guilt overwhelmed me, though I knew that in reality my presence would not have altered the course of her disease. The year was 1967. There were discussions among the senior physicians about the possibilities of peritoneal dialysis. However, Mary died before this treatment commenced.

It seems appropriate now, 50 years later, that I revisit these streptococcal related diseases to learn about their current frequencies and the discoveries related to their disease mechanisms that have been made in recent years.

Rheumatic Fever

In September 2001, Stollerman reviewed rheumatic fever. He emphasized that by the middle of the 20th century, data indicated that acute rheumatic fever followed infections caused by particularly virulent strains of Group A hemolytic streptococci. These strains formed mucoid colonies. These bacteria had large capsules with mucus-like coatings rich in hyaluronic acid and M protein, i.e. the M protein first described by Rebecca Lancefield.

Stollerman emphasized that the exact mechanism through which Group A beta-hemolytic streptococcal infections led to acute rheumatic fever in the post-infection period were still not known. However, there was evidence that particular components of the M protein stimulated antibody production in the host and that these antibodies also reacted with host tissues and caused their destruction. He reported that acute rheumatic fever outbreaks occurred during World War II and that specific group A beta-hemolytic streptococci subtypes rich in M protein were found to be responsible. He documented that in the 1970s there were few reports of acute rheumatic fever in the USA. However, in the 1980s acute rheumatic fever outbreaks were reported in Missouri, Utah and in the Rocky Mountain States.

The molecular structure of the M protein was determined through studies by Beachey et al. in 1979. Studies revealed that a specific portion of the M protein led to production of antibodies that reacted with several host tissues including joint linings (synovia) and heart valves. In some cases the antibodies reacted with skin components; in rare cases antibodies reacted with basal ganglia of the brain leading to a movement disorder, Sydenham's chorea. In cases in which significant damage to the heart valves occurs, chronic heart disease may result.

Further insights into the capsule and M protein of virulent group A beta-hemolytic streptococci were reported in 2013 by Lynskey et al. They noted that hyaluronic acid is a polymer composed of N-acetylglucosamine and glucuronic acid. Its formation is dependent on three enzymes: one responsible for production of glucuronic acid, another responsible for production of N-acetylglucosamine and a third enzyme, hyaluronic acid synthase, that acts to form polymers. Lynskey et al. discovered that a specific regulatory system exists in bacteria to control hyaluronic acid synthesis. One important regulatory gene is ROCA. It turns out that a specific defect in the ROCA gene leads bacteria to produce an excess of hyaluronic acid.

In the 1960s, the anti-streptolysin O test was used to diagnose streptococcal infections. Currently, other points of care diagnostics are used to rule out streptococcal pharyngitis. The rapid decline in occurrence of acute rheumatic fever in western countries coincided with antibiotic treatment of streptococcal infections and with improved socio-economic conditions.

In 2015, de Dassell et al. reviewed the incidence of rheumatic fever in developing countries. They noted that data on several countries was missing and that information on the global burden of rheumatic fever was thereby compromised. However, they estimated that the number of cases of rheumatic heart disease in the world exceeds 34 million. The prevalence of rheumatic heart disease is particularly high in Samoa and in the Solomon Islands, 89 cases per 1000 individuals in Samoa and 24 cases per 1000 in the Solomon Islands. Data from South Africa was not available for the 2015 de Dassell et al. report.

McLaren et al. (1975) reported that rheumatic heart disease occurred in 6 to 9 out of 1000 school children in Soweto, near Johannesburg, South Africa. In 2015, a study by Cilliers reported that the incidence of rheumatic heart disease in children in Soweto was 2 to 3 per thousand. In an echocardiographic screening of school children with average age of 12 years in the Lange and Bonteheuwel communities in Cape Town, South Africa, Mayosi (2014) reported in 2015 that the incidence of rheumatic heart disease was 20 cases per thousand. These authors reported that their echocardiographic studies in Jimma, Ethiopia revealed a rheumatic heart disease incidence of 31 per thousand.

Current point of care diagnostics to establish whether pharyngitis is due to pathogenic strains of group A beta-hemolytic streptococci include antibody tests and the use of DNA based studies to identify specific genes within those organisms. The DNA based studies make use of amplification methods such as polymerase chain reaction (PCR). There is a new methodology for DNA diagnosis that does not require a PCR machine and that can be done in a tube. This methodology is defined as LAMP; this is the abbreviation for loop mediated isothermal amplification (Tomlinson, 2014). It is based on the use of multiple primers that amplify a specific gene. If that gene is amplified in the LAMP reaction it indicates that presence of the specific organism.

The previously used standard method for detecting pathogenic organisms was the use of bacterial cultures. This method leads to delays in diagnosis, since culture requires 24–48 hours. It is important to note that some individuals are carriers of beta-hemolytic streptococci and may not necessarily have active infection.

Damage to Heart Valves and Further Complications

As young medical students in our preclinical years, we got to learn about a long term complication of rheumatic heart disease through the personal history of our professor of Microbiology. As a young man with damage to the mitral valve following rheumatic fever, he developed bacterial endocarditis. Bacterial foci on the damaged valve gave rise to emboli that passed from his heart to his brain. His prognosis was dire. Fortunately, he was able to receive treatment with penicillin from one of the first batches supplied to South Africa. He recovered from the acute infection but was left with a partial paralysis of one side of his body.

Bacterial Endocarditis in the 21st Century

Bacterial endocarditis, referred to currently in the USA as infective endocarditis, was reviewed in 2013 by Hoen et al. They reported that, in industrialized countries, the estimated annual incidence is 3 to 9 cases per 100,000 persons. They noted that the highest incidence was recorded in individuals with prosthetic heart valves, and in individuals with unrepaired cyanotic heart disease; rheumatic heart disease accounted for less than 10% of cases. Other conditions that predisposed to infective endocarditis included diabetes, human immune-deficiency disease and intravenous drug use. A number of cases fall into the category of healthcare associated endocarditis.

Hoen et al. reported that causative organisms are most frequently streptococci and staphylococci. Cerebral embolisms leading to hemorrhagic or ischemic stroke or to cerebral abscesses constitute the severest complications. They noted that large vegetative lesions on the heart valves are particularly found in cases of staphylococcal infections. The vegetations were revealed by echocardiography.

Post-streptococcal Glomerulonephritis

In a review of the pathogenesis of post-streptococcal glomerulonephritis by Rodriguez-Iturbo and Batsford in 2007, they noted that Wells published a paper in 1812 that described the latent period between scarlet fever and the appearance of dark urine. Reichel (1905) reported descriptions of glomerular lesions in fatal cases of nephritis that developed after scarlet fever. Futcher (1940) reported the occurrence of nephritis after streptococcal skin infections. Seegal and Earle (1941) reported that there were differences in the streptococcal strains that led to post-infection glomerulonephritis and strains that led to rheumatic fever. Subsequent studies proposed that immune complexes led to glomerulonephritis.

Rodriguez-Iturbo and Batsford (2007) reported that a likely pathogenic mechanism for post-streptococcal glomerulonephritis involves molecular mimicry. Specific streptococcal components likely induce antibodies that cross-react with specific renal structural components. There are reports indicating that streptococcal proteins share antigenic determinants with glomerulo-membrane proteins including laminin and vimentin. Poon King et al. (1993) reported that a kidney damaging strain of Streptococcus produced a protein defined as zSpeB. Rodriguez-Iturbo reported that rising titers of antibodies to zSpeB are the best indicators of post-streptococcal kidney damage. They concluded, however, that it is unlikely that a single pathogen is responsible for kidney damage.

Minodier et al. (2014) reported that in 2005 472,000 cases of post-streptococcal glomerulonephritis were reported in the world and 83% of cases occurred in developing countries.

Prevention of Rheumatic Heart Disease and Acute Glomerulonephritis in the Antibiotic Era

In their 2015 review of the occurrence of rheumatic heart disease following Group A beta-hemolytic streptococcal infections in developing countries, de Dassel et al. indicated that these organisms remain susceptible to treatment with benzathine penicillin G. A contra-indication to treatment is penicillin allergy.

Invasive Infections: New Diseases or Newly Recognized Diseases?

As specific disease due to Group A streptococci fade, others emerge. Invasive infection with group A streptococci, now referred to as *Streptococcus pyogenes*, have been associated with toxic shock syndrome (Davis *et al.*, 1980). This syndrome can also be caused by specific strains of *Staphylococcus*. The bacterial strains that cause toxic shock produce so called "super-antigen toxins" that result in polyclonal T cell activation and "storms" of cytokine production.

Toxic shock syndrome inducing infections may be related in some women to tampon use. Toxic shock syndrome may also occur secondarily to severe skin infections that occur after trauma, burns or surgery. This syndrome leads to severe fall in blood pressure and to multiple organ failure.

Antibiotic treatment with clindamycin is currently recommended in addition to removal of infected tissue and immunoglobulin infusions.

10 Tuberculosis

My most striking memories of tuberculosis patients in South Africa center on young children with tubercular meningitis. I have a distinct memory of a young child lying quite still in a cot whimpering rather than crying and only partly conscious. This child subsequently died and I attended the autopsy. The brain was covered in a thick greenish colored slime, likely composed of bacteria, white and red blood cells and degenerated tissue. It was this that deprived the child of life.

Van Well et al. published in 2009 a retrospective 20-year study of tuberculous meningitis in the Western Cape Province of South Africa. Their study included 554 patients, 82% of the patients studied were under five years of age. They reported that tuberculous meningitis in young children starts with non-specific symptoms. Patients were usually brought to the hospital only after manifestations such as impaired consciousness became evident. Other brain manifestations included motor deficits, evidence of cranial nerve dysfunction and partial paralysis. Detailed investigations often revealed evidence of tubercular lesions in the lungs. Diagnosis was made in part by finding CSF. The Mantoux tuberculin skin test was often positive.

Patient mortality was low, at 13% in the Van Well reported study. However, despite vigorous treatment with appropriate antibiotics children were often left with residual deficits. These included cognitive deficits, hearing or visual defects and in some cases motor functions were impaired.

Van Well et al. listed the following antibiotics used in treatment of tubercular meningitis during the course of the 20-year study: isoniazid, rifampicin, pyrazinamide and ethionamide. In addition, cortisone (prednisone) was given during the first month. Children with hydrocephalus also received diuretics. Patient outcomes were particularly poor in cases with HIV co-infection.

Some of my other memories of tuberculosis date from our microbiology class and the exciting information on an antibiotic, Streptomycin, that killed the *Mycobacterium tuberculosis* organism. Our professor spoke enthusiastically of the work of Doctor Rene Dubos on soil organisms that produce antibiotics and on the efforts of Doctor Waksman that led to availability of Streptomycin for clinical use.

The sixties and early seventies were times of optimism regarding treatment of tuberculosis. Although evidence emerged that *M. tuberculosis* became readily resistant to Streptomycin, other chemical compounds were developed that proved useful in treatment of tuberculosis. These included para-aminosalicylic acid (PAS), and Isoniazid. Later, ethambutol and rifampicin were added as effective treatment options. There was evidence that treatment with a combination of drugs defeated the organisms.

Bacillus Calmette and Guerin vaccine (BCG vaccine) was used to prevent tuberculosis in some countries, particularly in Europe after the Second World War. My own experience with BCG occurred in 1967. As a medical house officer in the Pediatrics department in Glasgow University working at the Queen Mother's Maternity hospital, one of my duties was to immunize all newborns with BCG skin injections.

BCG immunization was never adopted in the USA.

In 1995, an article in the Journal of Pediatrics (Colditz *et al.*) reviewed 1,264 different reports relating to BCG vaccination. They concluded that BCG vaccination of newborn infants reduced the risk of tuberculosis by 50%.

In a 2014 report, Mangtani *et al.* reported that BCG vaccine protection was greatest in environments where *M. tuberculosis* levels were low. They also reported that it was important to establish the individuals were not infected with tuberculosis at the time of immunization.

The WHO report (accessed January 2nd 2015) emphasized that BCG immunization is not recommended in cases that are positive for HIV, since in these cases BCG may result in significant complications.

Records indicate a decline in the incidence of tuberculosis in many countries in the 1960s and 1970s. However, the incidence remained high in socio-economically deprived areas. Tuberculosis has long been known to be a disease facilitated by adverse social conditions.

A History of Tuberculosis

Helen Bynum (2012) wrote a remarkable book on the history of tuberculosis. Bynum explored evidence that tuberculosis existed in pre-historic times. This evidence relates primarily to the specific lesions found on ancient skeletons. In addition, medical texts in ancient Greece from the time of Hippocrates had chapters on different forms of phthisis. Phthisis referred to excess secretions and impaired breathing. In the ancient texts, one form of phthisis including wasting of the body and the manifestation resembles the clinical features of tuberculosis.

Bynum noted that during the Renaissance period there was new interest in understanding the human body. Franciscus Sylvius (1614–1672) in the Netherlands described lesions in the lung, referred to as "tubercles", and their association with wasting consumption. Battista Morgagni (1682–1771) in Padua, Italy, described symptoms in patients and he also carried out post-mortems. He described tubercles in the lung and lymph glands.

Rene Laennec (1781–1826) in France pioneered detailed physical examination of patients. For examination of the chest he developed early forms of the stethoscope. Laennec also published detailed information on phthisis that began with military lesions, small seed-like lesions in the lung. He noted that these lesions increased in size and gave rise to tubercles. These tubercles were initially solid but later they liquefied. On coughing, patients would cough up liquid from these lesions and they would some-times cough up blood. Laennec also noted that in patients with lesions in the lung there were also often lesions in other organs.

In a chapter entitled "Consumption becomes Tuberculosis", Helen Bynum documented the remarkable work of Robert Koch that led up to his report to the Berlin Physiological Society on March 24th, 1882, "On the etiology of Tuberculosis".

The discovery that tuberculosis was caused by a germ led to measures in Britain to classify the disease as infectious and communicable, and to investigative measures to prevent the spread of the disease.

In the early part of the 20th century in Europe and in North America, sanatoria arose to isolate patients with tuberculosis and to establish physical conditions that facilitated natural cure of the disease.

Bynum noted that Calmette and Guerin in Paris worked for several decades to develop a weakened form of *Mycobacterium tuberculosis*.

In 1928, the BCG vaccine was used to inoculate children in Paris and in French Canada. Bynum recounted an unfortunate episode in 1931 when contaminated BCG vaccine caused death in children.

However, the BCG vaccination was actively adopted in Scandinavian countries. A clinical trial was carried out in Norway on two groups of nurses. The groups comprised one group who volunteered to receive the vaccine and another group who volunteered not to receive the vaccine. Later analysis revealed that nurses in the non-vaccinated group had six times the morbidity than was observed in the vaccinated group.

BCG vaccination of newborns was initiated in Scotland prior to its use in the rest of Britain. However, clinical studies carried out between 1953 and 1963 revealed convincing results of the efficacy of BCG vaccination. BCG vaccination was more widely used in Britain after 1963.

Bynum reviewed initiation of therapies for tuberculosis. The first antibiotic shown to kill *Mycobacterium tuberculosis* was Streptomycin, isolated from the soil fungus *Actinomyces griseus* by Waksman and Schatz in 1943. Following its isolation, the pharmaceutical company Merck initiated successful animal studies in 1944 and large-scale production of Streptomycin was then undertaken. Streptomycin was in use in patient therapy in 1946.

Other drugs to treat tuberculosis were soon developed. These included PAS related to salicylic acid and isoniazid related to nicotinic acid, utilized in the 1950s. Rifampicin was introduced in 1968. Additional anti-tuberculosis drugs have been introduced since then. Combination of therapies were found to be most efficacious in treatment of tuberculosis.

From the late 1940s, many countries introduced X-ray lung screening of the population in order to identify affected individuals and to initiate therapy and management.

Tuberculosis and Societal Conditions

In 1952 Rene Dubos, who had carried out important studies that laid the groundwork for anti-bacterial therapy of disease including tuberculosis published a book entitled "The White Plague". Rene's wife, Jean Dubos, who suffered from tuberculosis, is a co-author on the book. They noted evidence that in many countries the incidence of tuberculosis had begun to decline before the 1900s. They emphasized, "something happened in the mode of living in our civilization that rendered man more resistant to his ancient plague" (pp. 217–218).

It is important to emphasize the re-emergence of tuberculosis infections in recent decades. This occurred particularly in individuals whose immunological resistance was weakened by HIV/AIDS infections. Tuberculosis also occurs in individuals on the margins of society where living conditions and nutrition are marginal.

Tuberculosis Returns

In "The forgotten plague", Frank Ryan reported that from 1985 onward there was a progressive rise in the number of tuberculosis (TB) cases in New York. In 1992, the WHO reported that there was a dramatic increase in the number of TB cases in the developing world and in European countries including Switzerland, Denmark, the Netherlands, Sweden and the United Kingdom. The increase in TB incidence occurred at the same time that the incidence of HIV/AIDS increased. Ryan emphasized that all cases of TB do not also have HIV/AIDS, but that as TB increases in a population it can be more readily transmitted.

In a review of tuberculosis in Northern and Southern hemispheres, Hermans *et al.* (2015) analyzed reports of TB in Cape Town, South Africa, in New York and in London. Between 1910 and 1945, TB notifications in Cape Town were 450 per 100,000 individuals. Following chemotherapy introduction, in 1970 rates were 250 per 100,000. In 1995, rates had increased to 450 per 100,000. In 2010, rates were 850 per 100,000. Between 2009–2012, TB notifications in HIV negative individuals were 445 per 100,000 and in HIV positive individuals, rates were 6,338 per 100,000.

Tuberculosis and the Possibilities for Effective Vaccines

The earliest tuberculosis vaccine developed was BCG, that contains Bacillus Calmette Guerin (1927). This bacillus was derived from *Mycobacterium bovis* that causes tuberculosis in cattle. Calmette and Guerin subjected the organism to 230 passages and derived a weakened organism that could be used as a vaccine.

Weiner and Kaufman (2014) reported that the vaccine was predominantly used to prevent the serious consequences of tuberculosis infections in infants and children. These authors noted that in the early decades of the 20th century approximately 25% of infants who lived in households where there was an individual with active tuberculosis would die of tuberculosis. Institution in Europe of BCG vaccination of infants led to a rapid decrease in the death rates of infants and children. However, the protection afforded by BCG vaccination is transient and it does not protect adolescents and adults.

In the age of HIV, the WHO has reported that BCG immunization is not recommended in communities with high rates of HIV since it may be associated with complications (www.who.int/vaccine_safety/topics/bcg/immunocompromised/Dec_2006/en/).

The unique pathogenesis of tuberculosis complicates development of vaccines against the organism. Tuberculosis infection occurs most commonly through transmission of *Mycobacterium tuberculosis* (Mtb) bacteria from individuals with pulmonary tuberculosis, who have the organism in their sputum and secretions. It is known that the majority of individuals with active immune systems who are exposed to Mtb do not develop active tuberculosis disease (Weiner and Kaufman, 2014). They develop lesions referred to as granulomas in the lung, most often near the apex of the lung. The granulomas are rich in T lymphocytes and macrophage phagocytic cells that control the Mtb organism and limit their proliferation. In some cases with granulomas the bronchopulmonary lymph nodes may also manifest inflammation. This condition is known as latent tuberculosis. The granulomas are most often closed so that the individuals do not transmit Mtb. Individuals with latent tuberculosis are, however, immunologically sensitized to the Mtb organism. This sensitivity can be revealed by tuberculin skin tests or by a specific blood test that measures a protein known as interferon gamma release assay. There is, however, evidence that Mtb bacteria remain in the granulomas.

Salgame *et al.* (2015) reported that age has an important effect on whether latent tuberculosis will transform to active tuberculosis. Infants and children who have immature immune systems may not be able to control and limit the initial infection. High intensity exposure, e.g. the presence of high concentrations of Mtb in crowded, inadequately ventilated environments has been shown to lead to active disease even in adults. In addition, in immunodeficient individuals (children and adults), there is greater risk that primary infection will lead to active disease.

There is also evidence that individuals with latent tuberculosis may later transition to active tuberculosis, particularly if they become immunosuppressed through infection (with HIV for example) or through use of immune suppressive therapy (e.g. chemotherapy).

Maintenance of the latent tuberculosis status requires that the immune response is sufficient to inhibit proliferation of the Mtb present in granulomas. If the immune response fails to do this, the granuloma breaks down, the Mtb organism proliferates and spreads within the lung, and through the blood and lymphatic circulation to distant parts of the body.

It is also possible that individuals with latent tuberculosis may contract tuberculosis on renewed exposure to Mtb.

In 2015, the WHO reported that multiple Mtb vaccine strategies were being explored (http://www.who.int/immunization/research/development/tuberculosis/en/). These included development of vaccines given prior to Mtb exposure, development of vaccines for people who have latent tuberculosis with no evidence of clinical disease, and vaccines to be given to individuals apparently cured of tuberculosis through effective chemotherapy. The goal of immunization in the latter case is to prevent re-infection.

The 2015 WHO report states that sixteen different TB vaccines are in clinical trials. Five of these vaccines are based on whole-cell *Mycobacteria*. The remaining 11 vaccines are composed of specific subunits of Mtb. These include genes encoding the subunits cloned into recombinant viral vectors or specific Mtb subunit proteins produced through biotechnology and then combined with adjuvants that stimulate the immune response.

Some TB vaccines are also being developed based on modification of the BCG organism through use of genetic techniques. Mtb genes that encode specific antigenic proteins are cloned into BCG. Antigens frequently used in vaccines include Ag85A, Ag85B, ESAT6 and TB10-4 (Karp *et al.*, 2015). These investigators noted that the BCG organism has significant immune-stimulatory properties.

Karp *et al.* reported that the use of antibodies to treat tuberculosis has been dismissed since the Mtb organisms are primarily intra-cellular. They noted, however, that there was some evidence that humoral antibodies (antibodies in the blood stream and body fluids) could modify infection. However, further studies of this concept need to be carried out to confirm validity.

Biomarkers of Active Tuberculosis

A number of investigators have noted that there is need for development of biomarkers that could serve as a specific blood test to determine if an individual has transitioned from latent tuberculosis to active disease. This is important because sputum tests cannot always be relied on to indicate presence of Mtb. Weiner and Kaufman (2014) reported that research to develop biomarkers that will constitute signatures for active clinical tuberculosis was ongoing. Biomarkers being analyzed include cytokines and factors produced by cells of the immune system.

11 Tetanus

In 1963, when I was a final year medical student on rotation in the Pediatric inpatient service in the Academic Hospital in Pretoria, South Africa, the senior physician instructed me to enter very quietly into a room to observe a single patient there. He gave further instructions; there was to be no talking, no swift movements and the patient should not be touched. On entering the dimly lit room I observed a single tiny infant lying in a crib. The infant's hands were tightly clenched, his whole body was tensed and his back was slightly arched. The face muscles were tensed as though the infant was crying but he emitted no sounds. The senior physician then signaled to me to exit the room. He later explained that this was a case of neonatal tetanus. The patient had been brought in from a rural district and the physician suspected that the umbilical cord stump had likely been smeared with animal products, possibly with animal dung.

The image of that tiny rigid body with clenched fists has remained with me over many years. In 2016 I review current knowledge about neonatal tetanus, progress that has been made and the current extent of the problem in the world.

The spores of the bacterium *Clostridium tetani* are abundant in soil and in the gastro-intestinal tracts of vertebrates, including humans. The spores germinate under the low oxygen tissue conditions that exist in necrotic tissue. Spore germination and bacterial proliferation lead to production of the potent tetanus toxin. Neonatal tetanus results from unhygienic conditions of care of the umbilical cord of newborns.

Many reports include reviews of both neonatal and maternal tetanus. Maternal tetanus is defined as tetanus that occurs within six weeks of pregnancy, miscarriage or abortion. World Health Organization (WHO)

reports revealed that although neonatal and maternal tetanus were eliminated from developed countries more than half a century ago, in 1988
787,000 deaths of newborn infants from neonatal tetanus were reported;
in addition, many cases go unreported. A WHO plan to eliminate maternal
and neonatal tetanus was initiated in 1980. This plan includes provision
of education about hygienic practices and also immunization of women
with tetanus vaccine. In 2013, the WHO noted reports of death of 49,000
infants due to neonatal tetanus.

Maternal and neonatal tetanus has now been eliminated from many
more countries, including China, South Africa and parts of India. Thwaites
et al. (2015) reported that 24 countries had not yet eliminated maternal
and neonatal tetanus. It still occurs in countries in Sub-Saharan Africa, in
Pakistan and some states bordering Pakistan, in some states in India and
in some Pacific Island countries including New Guinea.

It is important to note that natural disasters, that include flooding,
frequently also lead to open wounds. Such open wounds are associated
with increased risk of tetanus in unimmunized persons.

There is now evidence that the tetanus toxin is produced by an
intracellular plasmid that is present in the *Clostridium tetani* bacillus. This
toxin is released as bacteria die. Roper *et al.* (2007) reported that the toxin
binds to peripheral neurons. The toxin is also transported through the blood
and the lymphatic system and it binds to distal neurons. The main action
of the tetanus toxin is to impair the function of inhibitory neurons. This
lack of inhibitory function leads to unopposed excitation of motor neurons
and results in muscle rigidity. Physical, auditory or visual stimuli precipitate
painful muscle spasms. The extreme muscle spasms prevent infants from
sucking and feeding. In addition, spasms of the respiratory muscles impair
breathing. Thwaites *et al.* reported that the autonomic nervous system is
also impaired, leading to increased noradrenaline and adrenaline, and to
cardio-vascular abnormalities including arrhythmias and blood pressure
abnormalities. The mortality rates in maternal and neonatal tetanus are
very high. Hospital treatment includes use of antibiotics, administration
of anti-convulsive agents, use of tetanus anti-toxin and where possible
assisted ventilation.

The key prevention of maternal and neonatal tetanus is achieved
through improved perinatal care and immunization of women, including
pregnant women. There is evidence that maternal anti-tetanus antibodies

pass to the fetus. However, in women infected with HIV or malaria, passage of antibodies to the fetus may be impaired. Thwaite *et al.* report that, in places where environmental conditions predispose to maternal and neonatal tetanus, it is advisable also for women who have received immunization in childhood (most often with Diphtheria, Pertussis tetanus DPT vaccine) to have tetanus vaccine booster immunization as adults.

12 Viral Infections that May Lead to Cancer

(a) Hepatitis Viruses and Hepatoma

As a medical student working in 1962 in the internal medicine service at the Pretoria Academic Hospital in Pretoria, I was frequently assigned to interview and examine middle aged or relatively young African men who were in great discomfort due to very marked swelling and distension of their abdomens. Several of these men had traveled to the hospital from distant rural regions.

The abdominal swelling in these patients was in part due to the accumulation of large quantities of fluid in the abdominal cavity, a condition referred to as ascites. Abdominal swelling was also due to enlargement of their livers. Under the supervision of senior physicians, I carried out a procedure to remove the excess fluid. Following this procedure, a patient would feel more comfortable and was grateful. However, I had to let him know that relief would be only temporary and fluid would slowly accumulate again. Following removal of the ascetic fluid, abdominal palpation revealed the extent to which the liver was enlarged, hardened and sometimes of abnormal shape.

These patients had primary hepatocellular cancer, also referred to as hepatoma, and their prognoses were grave. There was no specific treatment.

To try to learn more about hepatoma, I visited the Pathology department and consulted a mentor, Dr. Pepler. He graciously allowed me to view microscopic slides of hepatocellular carcinoma prepared following autopsies on previous patients. Histology analyses revealed that there was frequently evidence of underlying liver cirrhosis in patients with hepatoma. I also searched the literature for information on possible causes of hepatoma. In the literature, causes of cirrhosis were described and these often included exposure to harmful substances. A few reports indicated that exposure to foods contaminated with mold represented an important risk factor.

As an aside, I wrote an essay that described histological findings in the few cases of hepatoma that I had examined, and I summarized information from the literature on possible risk factors and submitted this to the South African Cancer Society as an entry to a competition open to medical students. I received a financial award and the funds were very useful as I purchased books and supplies for my final year in medical school.

In later years, I returned to a study on hepatomas, revealing that in many hepatomas the patterns of expression of human alcohol dehydrogenase (ADH) enzymes changed and that the fetal forms of the enzyme became the predominantly expressed form. This was of interest, since it was known that hepatomas manifested altered expression with decreased expression of albumin and increased expression of alpha fetoprotein.

It was only later, in the 1970s, that the importance of the newly discovered Hepatitis B virus in etiology of hepatoma was reported through studies carried out primarily in the USA and in England.

Discovery of Hepatitis B Virus

Discovery of a key agent in the causation of hepatitis and liver cancer emerged through research in population genetics and though use of immunological techniques. Alter, Blumberg and co-workers undertook research to identify genetic variation in human blood proteins; they studied blood samples derived from individuals in different countries. The key approach was to utilize immunological techniques to search for unusual blood proteins (antigens) present in the serum of specific individuals, that reacted with antibodies present in the serum of other individuals who had received multiple blood transfusions.

During the course of their research they identified a specific antigen in the blood of an individual from Australia that reacted with antibodies present in the blood from a patient who had received multiple blood transfusions to treat hemophilia. The antigen was labeled the Australia antigen, AuAg (Alter and Blumberg, 1966). In subsequent studies, the AuAg was found to react with antibodies in the blood of patients who had previously had hepatitis.

Serendipitously, around the same time Prince at the New York Blood Center identified a specific antigen in the blood of hepatitis patients and he labeled this antigen SH. In 1968, Prince reported that the SH antigen and the Australia antigen AuAg were closely related or identical.

These discoveries led to a series of experiments to characterize the Australia antigen more fully and to determine its origins. Electron microscopic studies initially revealed that the AuAg was a protein. However, in more detailed electron microscopic studies, Dane et al. (1970) determined that the AuAg complexes contained not only small protein particles but also larger virus-like particles. The virus-like particles became known as Dane particles.

Further studies of the virus-like particles revealed that they contained a specific enzyme that could synthesis DNA, a DNA polymerase. In 1978, the DNA synthesized by the virus-like Dane particles was cloned and sequenced and became known as the Hepatitis B virus. Availability of the purified virus and its sequence improved diagnostic testing of patient samples and also facilitated screening of blood to be used for donation.

Hepatitis B Virus and Hepatoma

Szmuness (1978) reported that chronic hepatitis infection led to increased incidence of hepatocellular carcinoma (hepatoma). In studies on cultured hepatoma cells and in studies on hepatoma tumors, the hepatitis B virus (HBV) was found to have integrated into the host chromosomes.

There is evidence that a specific protein produced by the integrated HBV DNA deregulates the host genome and activates expression of genes that promote tumor formation (Hohne et al., 1990).

Development of an HBV Vaccine

In a review of the virology of Hepatitis B, Gerlich (2013) noted that the sequencing of the HBV genome and cloning of the HBV genome or genome fragments into yeast enable the production of large quantities of the major HBV proteins, and this facilitated vaccine production. The HBsAg protein is used to produce the vaccine. More recent studies have revealed that it is also useful in producing vaccines to include HBV material upstream of the DNA sequence that encodes HBs Ag.

Successes Achieved with HBV Vaccine

Taiwan introduced HBV vaccination of children in 1984. A report in 2009 by Chang et al. revealed a significant drop in the incidence of hepatocellular carcinoma in Taiwan.

In 2013, Kane et al. noted that the majority of liver disease and cirrhosis in China was due to Hepatitis B infection. They reported results of a GAVI Alliance hepatitis immunization project initiated in China in 2002. Free HBV vaccination and safe injection practices were made available in 12 western provinces of China and in 10 provinces in central China where the poverty index was high. Kane et al. reported that, as a result of this immunization project, the carrier rate for hepatitis B in children five years of age fell from 10% to 1%.

Hepatitis B Worldwide

A WHO report updated in 2015 noted that Hepatitis B infections remain important problems in East Asia and in sub-Saharan Africa, where 5–10% of individuals in the population have chronic hepatitis B infection. High rates of this infection also occur in Eastern Europe, in the Middle-East and in India.

There is evidence that HBV infection spreads horizontally from mothers to children. In children, hepatitis B infection often becomes chronic. Horizontal infection transmission can also occur from infected children to uninfected children. In addition, individuals may become infected through exposure to infected blood, during medical and surgical procedures and during tattooing.

In acute and in chronic infection, both HBsAg antigen and HB core antigen (HBc) antigen can be detected. Another antigen, HBeAg, also occurs in individuals with severe infection. The WHO report noted that persistence of HBsAg is a marker for chronic disease and is associated with hepatocellular carcinoma. Amponsah-DaCosta et al. (2014) reported that immunization increased the presence of antibodies to HBV and the levels of immunity to HBV infections, particularly in individuals negative for HIV/AIDS infections.

Hepatitis B and Hepatitis C in Hepatocellular Carcinoma

In a report on hepatocellular carcinoma in developing countries, Kew (2012) documented that in resource-poor countries children frequently did not receive a full course of hepatitis B vaccine. Kew stressed the importance of both hepatitis B and hepatitis C in infections and the contamination of food with aflatoxin fungus in the etiology of hepatocellular carcinoma.

Kew noted the importance of measurement of blood alpha-fetoprotein in diagnosis of hepatocellular carcinoma. Even in 2012, patients in South Africa with hepatocellular carcinoma usually presented late in the course of their disease.

The prognosis of patients with hepatocellular carcinoma remains poor. However, one chemotherapeutic agent (Sorafenib) has proved useful in decreasing tumor size. Kew emphasized that in resource-poor countries the cost of treatment with Sorafenib limits access and use.

Hepatocellular Carcinoma and Hepatitis B and C Viruses Worldwide

In 2015, de Martel *et al.* reported results of studies in 119,000 cases of hepatocellular carcinoma. Their studies revealed that in Europe and in America there were more hepatitis C associated cases of hepatocellular carcinoma than hepatitis B virus associated cases, and there were also substantial increases in the number of associated cases of hepatocellular carcinoma in Brazil and Germany in the years after 2000. In Asian and African countries, hepatitis B virus associated cases of hepatocellular carcinoma predominated.

Attempts to Control Hepatitis C Virus Infections

Hepatitis C virus is transferred through blood, body fluids and the use of inadequately sterilized medical equipment. As of 2016, no vaccines were available to prevent hepatitis C infection.

Houghton (2009) reported that identification of the hepatitis C virus was an arduous process. The hepatitis C virus turned out to be a 10,000 nucleotide single stranded RNA virus that is extra-chromosomal in host cells.

A number of direct acting anti-retroviral drugs were identified that are successful in eliminating the virus. However, these drugs are costly and costs may prohibit their use. Drugs active against hepatitis C virus include protease inhibitors and nucleoside inhibitors.

Hepatitis C viral infection often co-occurs with HIV/AIDS infection. There is evidence that intact uncompromised T lymphocyte responses are important in clearance of hepatitis C virus (Major, 2016).

Mycotoxins

Kew (2012) referred to the possible implications of aflatoxin, a mycotoxin that is a likely risk factor in the development of hepatic cancer. I decided, therefore, to go in search of information on mycotoxins.

Mycotoxins are metabolites produced by fungi that colonize specific cereal crops. *Aspergillus* fungi produce aflatoxins. Fungi belonging to the genus *Fusarium* produce fumonisin. Specific types of *Penicillium* fungi produce ochratoxin.

Maize can be infected with all three types of fungi. Wheat, barley and oats can be infected by *Aspergillus* and *Penicillium*. *Aspergillus* can also infect tree nuts and peanuts (Wu *et al.*, 2014).

Studies carried out in different parts of the world have investigated the relationship of aflatoxins to hepatocellular carcinoma. Many studies have been carried out in China and in South Africa. Aflatoxin-derived metabolites have been shown to reach high levels in men with liver cancer. There is also evidence that aflatoxin exposure acts synergistically with hepatitis B virus in causing liver cancer (Sun *et al.*, 1999). Acute exposures to high levels of aflatoxins lead to acute liver damage.

(b) Human Papilloma Virus, Cervical and other Cancers

One of the main problems encountered in Gynecological Services in South Africa in the 1960s was cervical cancer and it remains a significant problem worldwide. In 2012, Forman *et al.* reported, based on worldwide statistics gathered in 2008, that cervical cancer was the fourth most common cause of cancer deaths in females. They noted further that there was strong association between cervical cancer incidence and stage of economic development of countries. They reported that 88% of cervical cancer deaths occurred in less developed regions of the world.

During the 1970s, extensive work and classification on papilloma viruses was carried out; research on papilloma viruses was facilitated by studies of Klug and Finch (1968). In the late 1970s, histologic and electron microscopic studies revealed that the papilloma viruses were present in the abnormal precancerous dysplastic cells present in cervical smears (Lavert, 1979). In 1983, Durst and members of the zur Hausen team reported that papilloma virus DNA occurred in cancer biopsy samples. In the years following their report, human papilloma virus has been shown to be the predominant cause of squamous cell carcinoma of the cervix, the predominant form of cervical cancer.

Harald zur Hausen received the Nobel Prize in Physiology and Medicine in 2008 for his discovery of the role of papilloma viruses in cancer.

Human papilloma viruses have also been shown to play important roles in cancers of the anogenital regions in men and women and in cancers of the mouth and throat (Marur et al., 2010).

Studies have revealed that specific proteins produced by papilloma virus interact with and inhibit host proteins that normally act as tumor suppressors.

Development of a Vaccine that Induces Immunity to Human Papilloma Viruses

A vaccine against human papilloma viruses (HPV) was developed in 2006. The approved HPV vaccine is prepared from protein shells of HPV16 and HPV18 and does not contain HPV DNA. The vaccine induces antibodies against HPV. Three spaced doses of vaccine are recommended and immunization should ideally commence in the pre-adolescent years (WHO reports accessed February 2016).

(b) Herpes 8 Virus and Kaposi Sarcoma

In South Africa in the 1960s, we frequently met with patients who had unusual skin lesions, raised nodules that had a purplish color. Similar lesions sometimes occurred on mucous membranes. We learned that these lesions were defined as Kaposi sarcoma.

In 1994, Chang *et al.* determined that the Kaposi sarcoma lesions were due to infection with a particular virus, Herpes 8. It has also become evident that immunodeficiency plays an important role in development of these lesions (Radu and Pantanowitz, 2013). The immunodeficiency may have a number of different causes. Kaposi sarcoma lesion may occur in individuals with HIV/Aids; they may also occur in individuals who receive immunosuppressive therapy following transplantation. Kaposi sarcoma has also been reported in rare cases of immunodeficiency due to mutations in genes that control elements of the immune system.

There is evidence that the Kaposi sarcoma lesions regress during anti-retroviral treatment.

13 HIV/AIDS

My own experience of the impact of HIV/AIDS is South Africa related to children. In 2008, I visited an orphanage for infants and children whose mothers were severely affected by AIDS and were unable to take care of them. No other family members had come forward to care for the children. Some of the orphans were also positive for HIV and were receiving treatment. On another occasion, while on a visit to the Chris Hani hospital in Soweto near Johannesburg, I was taken to a clinic for Pediatric HIV/AIDS patients; many of the children were very thin and seemed much debilitated. I noticed that many children were brought to the clinic by grandmothers and was told that many of the children lived with their grandparents, since parents were not available to take care of them.

Currently, anti-retroviral therapies are effective in controlling HIV/AIDS. However, life-long treatments with several drugs are required. In addition, side effects of the drugs occur.

References

Alter HJ, Blumberg BS. (1966). Further studies on a "new" human isoprecipitin system (Australia antigen). *Blood* 27(3):297–309. PMID:5930797.

Amponsah-Dacosta E, Lebelo RL, Rakgole JN, *et al.* (2014). Evidence for a change in the epidemiology of hepatitis B virus infection after nearly two decades of universal hepatitis B vaccination in South Africa. *Med Virol* 86(6):918–24. doi: 10.1002/jmv.23910.

Beachey EH, Stolleman GH, Johnson RH *et al.* (1979). Human immune response to immunization with a structurally defined polypeptide fragment of streptococcal M protein. *J Exp Med* 150(4):862–877. PMID:390084.

Bynum H. (2012). *Spitting Blood. The History of Tuberculosis.* Oxford University Press.

Calmette A, Guerin C, Boquet A, *et al.* (1927). *La vaccination préventive contre la tuberculose par le "BCG.".* Paris: Masson et cie.

Cilliers AM. (2015). Rheumatic fever and rheumatic heart disease in Africa. *S Afr Med J* **105(5):**361–2. doi: 10.7196/samj.9433. PMID:26242662.

Colditz GA, Berkey CS, Mosteller F, *et al.* (1995). The efficacy of bacillus Calmette-Guerin vaccination of newborns and infants in the prevention of tuberculosis: meta-analyses of the published literature. *Pediatrics* **96(1 Pt 1):** 29–35. PMID:7596718.

Chang MH, You SL, Chen CJ, *et al.* (2009). Decreased incidence of hepatocellular carcinoma in hepatitis B vaccinees: a 20-year follow-up study. *J Natl Cancer Inst* **101(19):**1348–55. doi: 10.1093/jnci/djp288. PMID:19759364.

Chang Y, Cesarman E, Pessin MS, *et al.* (1994). Identification of herpesvirus-like DNA sequences in AIDS-associated Kaposi's sarcoma. *Science* **266(5192):**1865–9. PMID:7997879.

Dale JB, Beachey EH. (1985). Epitopes of Streptococcal M protein shared with cardiac myosin Epitopes of streptococcal M proteins shared with cardiac myosin. *J Exp Med* **162(2):**583–591. PMCID: PMC2187745.

Dane DS, Cameron CH, Briggs M. (1970). Virus-like particles in serum of patients with Australia-antigen-associated hepatitis. *Lancet* **1(7649):**695–8. PMID:4190997.

Davis JP, Chesney PJ, Wand PJ, LaVenture M. (1980). Toxic-shock syndrome: epidemiologic features, recurrence, risk factors, and prevention. *N Engl J Med* **303(25):**1429–35. PMID:7432401.

de Dassel JL, Ralph AP, Carapetis JR. (2015). Controlling acute rheumatic fever and rheumatic heart disease in developing countries: are we getting closer? *Curr Opin Pediatr* **27(1):**116–23. doi: 10.1097/MOP.0000000000000164. PMID:25490689.

de Martel C, Maucort-Boulch D, Plummer M, Franceschi S. (2015). World-wide relative contribution of hepatitis B and C viruses in hepatocellular carcinoma. *Hepatology* **62(4):**1190–200. doi: 10.1002/hep.27969. PMID:26146815.

Dubos RJ, Dubos J. (1952). *The White Plague: Tuberculosis, Man and Society.* Little Brown and Company, Boston pp.217–218.

Dürst M, Gissmann L, Ikenberg H, zur Hausen H. (1983). A papillomavirus DNA from a cervical carcinoma and its prevalence in cancer biopsy samples from different geographic regions. *Proc Natl Acad Sci USA* **80(12):**3812–5. PMID:6304740.

Forman D, De Martel C, Lancey CJ, *et al.* (2012). Global burden of human papillomavirus and related diseases. *Vaccine* **30(5):** F12–23. PMID: 23199955. Doi: 10.1016/j.vaccine 2012.07.055.

Futcher PH. (1940). Glomerular nephritis following infections of the skin. *Arch Int Med* **65(6):**1192–1210.

Gerlich WH. (2013). Medical virology of hepatitis B: how it began and where we are now. *Virol J* **10:**239. doi: 10.1186/1743-422X-10-239. PMID:23870415.

Griffith E. (1978). The significance of Pneumococcal types. *J Hyg* (Lond) **27(2):**113–59. PMID: 20474956.

Hermans S, Horsburgh CR Jr, Wood R. (2015). A century of tuberculosis epidemiology in the northern and southern hemisphere: the differential impact of control interventions. *PLoS One* **10(8):**e0135179. doi: 10.1371/journal.pone.0135179. PMID:26288079.

Hills E, Laverty CR (1979). Electron microscope detection of papilloma virus particles in selected koilocytotic cells in a routine cervical smear. *Acta Cytol* **23(1):**53–6. PMID:219647.

Hoen B, Duval X. (2013). Clinical practice. Infective endocarditis. *N Engl J Med* **368(15):**1425–33. doi: 10.1056/NEJMcp1206782. PMID:23574121.

Hohne M, Schaefer S, Seifer M, *et al.* (1990). Malignant transformation of immortalized transgenic hepatocytes after transfection with hepatitis virus DNA. *EMBO J* **9:**1137–45. PMID:23233.

Houghton M. (2009). Discovery of the hepatitis C virus. *Liver Int* **29 Suppl 1:**82–8. doi: 10.1111/j.1478-3231.2008.01925.x. PMID:19207970.

Kane MA, Hadler SC, Lee L, *et al.* (2013). The inception, achievements, and implications of the China GAVI Alliance Project on Hepatitis B Immunization. *Vaccine* **31 Suppl 9:**J15–20. doi: 10.1016/j.vaccine.2013.03.045. PMID:24331015.

Karp CL, Wilson CB, Stuart LM. (2015). Tuberculosis vaccines: barriers and prospects on the quest for a transfomative tool. *Immunol Rev* **264(1):**363–81. doi: 10.111/imr.12270. PMID:25703572.

Kew MC. (2012). Hepatocellular carcinoma in developing countries: Prevention, diagnosis and treatment. *World J Hepatol* **4(3):**99–104. doi: 10.4254/wjh.v4.i3.99. PMID:22489262.

Klug A, Finch JT. (1968). Structure of viruses of the papilloma-polyoma type. IV Analysis of tilting experiments in the electron microscope. *J Mol Bio* **14: 31(1):** 1–12. PMID: 4295242.

Lancefield RC. (1933). A serological differentiation of human and other groups of hemolytic streptococci. *J Exp Med* **57(4):**571–95. PMID:19870148.

Lynskey NN, Goulding D, Gierula M, *et al.* (2013). RocA truncation underpins hyper-encapsulation, carriage longevity and transmissibility of serotype M18 group A streptococci. *PLoS Pathog* **9(12):**e1003842. doi: 10.1371/journal.ppat.1003842. PMID:24367267.

Major ME. (2016). Hepatitis C: new clues to better vaccines? *Gut* **65(1):**4–5. doi: 10.1136/gutjnl-2015-309829. PMID:26092844.

Mangtani P, Abubakar I, Ariti C, *et al.* (2014). Protection by BCG vaccine against tuberculosis: a systematic review of randomized controlled trials. *Clin Infect Dis* **58(4):**470–80. doi: 10.1093/cid/cit790. PMID:24336911.

Marur S, D'Souza G, Westra WH, Forastiere AA. (2010). HPV-associated head and neck cancer: a virus-related cancer epidemic. *Lancet Oncol* **11(8):**781–9. doi: 10.1016/S1470-2045(10)70017-6. PMID:20451455.

Mayosi BM. (2014). The challenge of silent rheumatic heart disease. *Lancet Glob Health* **2(12):**e677–8. doi: 10.1016/S2214-109X(14)70331-6. PMID: 25433614.

McCarty M. (1987). Rebecca Craighill Lancefield: January 5, 1895-March 3, 1981. *Biogr Mem Natl Acad Sci* **57:**227–46.

McLaren MJ, Hawkins DM, Koornhof HJ, *et al.* (1975). Epidemiology of rheumatic heart disease in black schoolchildren of Soweto, Johannesburg. *Br Med J* **23**;3(5981): 474–8. PMID: 1156827.

Minodier P, LaPorte R, Miramont S (2014). Epidemiology of Streptococcus pyogenes infections in developing countries. *Arch Pediatr* **21 Suppl 2:** S69–72. doi: 10.1016/S0929-693X(14)72263-8. Epub 2014 Nov 13.

Poon-King R, Bannan J, Viteri A, *et al.* (1993). Identification of an extracellular plasmin binding protein from nephritogenic streptococci. *J Exp Med* **178(2):** 759–63. PMID:8340765.

Prince AM. (1968). Relation of Australia and SH antigens. *Lancet* **2(7565):**462–3. PMID:4174193.

Radu O, Pantanowitz L. (2013). Kaposi sarcoma. *Arch Pathol Lab Med* **137(2):** 289–94. doi: 10.5858/arpa.2012-0101-RS. PMID:23368874.

Reichel H. (1905). Uber Nephritis bei Scharlach. *Z Heil* **6:**72–78.

Rodríguez-Iturbe B, Batsford S. (2007). Pathogenesis of poststreptococcal glomerulonephritis a century after Clemens von Pirquet. *Kidney Int* **71(11):** 1094–104. PMID:17342179.

Roper MH, Vandelaer JH, Gasse FL. (2007). Maternal and neonatal tetanus. *Lancet* **370(9603):**1947–59. PMID:17854885.

Ryan F. (1992). *The Forgotten Plague: How the Battle against Tuberculosis was Won and Lost.* Little, Brown and Company Boston, New York, London.

Salgame P, Geadas C, Collins L, *et al.* (2015). Latent tuberculosis infection-- Revisiting and revising concepts. *Tuberculosis (Edinb)* **95(4):**373–84. doi: 10. 1016/j.tube.2015.04.003. PMID:26038289.

Seegal D, Earle DP. (1941). A consideration of certain biological differences between glomerulonephritis and rheumatic fever. *Am J Med Sci* **201:**528–539.

Stollerman GH. (2001). Rheumatic fever in the 21st century. *Clin Infect Dis* **33(6):**806–14. PMID:11512086.

Sun S, Lu P, Gail MH, *et al.* (1999). Increased risk of hepatocellular carcinoma in male hepatitis surface antigen carriers with chronic hepatitis who have de-tectable urinary aflatoxin metabolite M1. *Hepatology* **30(2):** 379–383. PMID: 10421643.

Szmuness W. (1979). Hepatocellular carcinoma and the hepatitis B virus: evidence for a causal association. *Prog Med Virol* **24:**40–69. PMID:212785.

Thwaites CL, Beeching NJ, Newton CR. (2015). Maternal and neonatal tetanus. *Lancet* **385(9965):**362–70. doi: 10.1016/S0140-6736(14)60236-1. PMID:25149223.

Tomlinson J. (2013). In-field diagnostics using loop-mediated isothermal amplification. *Methods Mol Biol* **938:**291–300. doi: 10.1007/978-1-62703-089-2_25. PMID:22987425.

van Well GT, Paes BF, Terwee CB, *et al.* (2009). Twenty years of pediatric tuberculous meningitis: a retrospective cohort study in the western cape of South Africa. *Pediatrics* **123(1):**e1–8. PMID:19367678.

Waksman SA, Schatz A. (1943). Strain specificity and production of antibiotic substances. *Proc Natl Acad Sci USA* **29(2):**74–9. PMID:16588605.

Weiner J 3rd, Kaufman SH. (2014) Recent advances toward tuberculosis control: vaccines and biomarkers. *J Inter Med* **275(5):**467–480. doi: 10.1111/joim.12212. PMID:24635488.

Wells CD. (1812). Observations on the dropsy which succeeds scarlet fever. *Trans Soc Imp Med Chir Knowledge* **3:**167–186.

World Health Organization WHO: Maternal and Neonatal Tetanus (MNT) elimination http://www.who.int/immunization/diseases/MNTE_initiative/en/ Sep 7, 2015

WHO: Hepatitis B (Fact sheet No 204). Updated July 2015. www.who.int/mediacentre/factsheets/fs204/en/

WHO: Human papillomavirus and HPV vaccines: a review http://www.who.int/bulletin/volumes/85/9/06-038414/en/

WHO: Safety of human papillomavirus vaccines — World Health Organization www.who.int/vaccine_safety/topics/hpv/en/

Wu F, Groopman JD, Pestka JJ. (2014). Public health impacts of foodborne mycotoxins. *Annu Rev Food Sci Technol* **5:**351–72. doi: 10.1146/annurev-food-030713-092431. PMID:24422587.

Young BC, Levine RJ, Karumanchi SA. (2010). Pathogenesis of preeclampsia. *Annu Rev Pathol* **5:**173–92 doi.1146/annrev-pathol-12180n-102149. PMID: 20078220.

PART IV

Infections, Therapy and Prevention

14 The Golden Age of Antibiotics, and Has it Passed?

In recent years, and particularly in 2015, there have been many reports on antibiotic resistant micro-organisms. In 2015, several national and international incentives were established to promote discovery of new antibiotics to add to the clinical pipeline. In 2016, Brown and Wright noted: "Lessons from the history of antibiotic discovery and fresh understanding of antibiotic action and the cell biology of microorganisms have the potential to deliver twenty-first century medicines that are able to control infection in the resistance era."

The Golden Age

The Golden Age of antibiotic discovery and development for clinical use occurred approximately between the early 1940s and the mid-1970s (Chopra, 2013). Coates *et al.* (2011) reported that twenty new classes of antibiotics were marketed between 1940 and 1962 and that since then only two new classes have become available for clinical use. An overview of classes of antibiotics and their function is available at www.compoundchem.com. In this section I discuss the development of antibiotics. It is important to note that many of these antibiotics in the classes described were isolated from fungi or bacteria. Chemical analyses were critical to define the structure of the antibiotics. Subsequently, chemical modifications of antibiotics could be carried out to produce variant forms of specific antibiotics. In relatively few cases were antibiotics synthesized *de novo* in the laboratory.

The first chemotherapeutic agent to treat infections, Sulfonamide, became available in the late 1930s. Penicillin and related beta-lactam antibiotics became available in the 1940s, after 1942. Beta-lactam antibiotics include penicillin, amoxicillin, methicillin and cephalosporin. Beta-lactam antibiotics impact synthesis of bacterial cell walls. Some bacteria developed resistance to these antibiotics through production of lactamase. This resistance was overcome to a significant extent by addition of lactamase inhibitors to beta-lactam antibiotics.

The aminoglycoside class of antibiotics (including streptomycin, kanamycin and neomycin) became available later in the 1940s. Aminoglycosides inhibit protein synthesis in bacteria. Chloramphenicol, that also inhibits bacterial protein synthesis, became available in the 1950s but its use was limited by toxic effects.

Tetracyclines (developed in the 1950s) are composed of hydrocarbon rings and this class includes tetracycline, doxycycline and oxycycline, that all inhibit bacterial protein synthesis. The macrolide antibiotics, also developed in the 1950s, contain 14, 15 or 16 membered macrolide rings. The macrolide class of antibiotics includes erythromycin, clarithromycin and azithromycin and they inhibit bacterial protein synthesis.

In the 1960s, the Glycopeptide class of antibiotics was developed. These antibiotics have a particularly complex structure, with carbohydrates linked to peptides. They include vancomycin and teicoplanin (Targocid). These antibiotics are used to treat methicillin resistant *Staphylococcus aureus* infections. Glycopeptide antibiotics inhibit bacterial cell wall synthesis.

The Ansamycin class of antibiotics was developed in the 1960s. They are composed of aromatic rings bridged by aliphatic chains. The class includes geldanamycin, rifamycin and naphthanamycin. These antibiotics inhibit RNA synthesis. They also have antiviral activity. Rifampin used to treat tuberculosis and leprosy was developed through chemical modifications of rifamycin.

The Streptogramin class of antibiotics was developed in the 1960s and is composed of two structurally different antibiotics that act synergistically. These are Pristinamycin IA and Pristinamycin IIa; they are used to treat gram positive bacterial infections.

In the 1970s, the Quinolone class of antibiotics was developed. They are comprised of fused aromatic rings attached to carboxylic acid and fluoride is often attached to an aromatic ring. Quinolone antibiotics include ciprofloxacin, and levofloxacin. They act by impairing DNA synthesis. Resistance to these antibiotics readily develops.

Antibiotic classes developed in the 1980s included Oxazolidinones (linezolid, cycloserine and posizolid) and Lipopeptides, lipids bound to peptides (daptomycin and surfactin).

A History of Penicillin Discovery

Recently, I read again the exciting history of penicillin discovery, "The mold in Dr. Florey's coat", written by Eric Lax.

The capacity of the mold *Penicillium notatum* to destroy bacteria was reported by Alexander Fleming in 1928. However, intense efforts to identify the antibacterial component of the *Penicillium* mold started only in 1939, when Boris Chaim and Norman Heatley in Oxford applied intense efforts to the problem.

Their ability to find minimal funding for the project was somewhat facilitated by the prospect that injuries from the Second World War were likely to be severe; if individuals survived injury, infections of wounds would likely compromise survival. Obtaining ongoing funding was extremely difficult.

For their studies, Florey and his team were able to obtain a *Penicillium notatum* culture in Oxford. Equipment for culturing organisms was hard to come by and the team used whatever utensils they could lay hands on, including biscuit tins. Extraction of the active compound required filtration of culture fluids, facilitated at one point by a donation of parachute silk. Filtered culture was then extracted with ether or amyl acetate followed by steam distillation to separate solvents from penicillin. Chromatography was then carried out and this was followed by freeze drying. Equipment had to be built from any available material or utensils. Lax indicates that Norman Heatley was a genius at designing and building makeshift equipment.

The active component, penicillin, which could kill bacteria in culture, was tested for toxicity and bacterial killing ability in mice and rabbits.

In August 1940, Chain, Florey and team had a two-page article published in the medical journal Lancet with the title: "Penicillin as a chemotherapeutic agent".

Lax recorded in his book that on January 27th, 1941 a toxicity test of penicillin was carried out on a woman with terminal cancer. The patient gave consent to the test though she knew it would not help her condition. The patient stated that she was "rather proud to help in this important test". Two tests of penicillin were carried out. The first test led the patient to experience chills and the sample of penicillin was found to contain py-rogens. A second test was carried out using a sample of penicillin that had undergone further purification by chromatography. That solution did not cause the patient to have chills. High levels of penicillin were found in the patient's blood and penicillin was secreted in the urine. Subsequent tests were carried out in Oxford on patients who had severe infections and the efficacy of penicillin in killing infection-causing bacteria in patients without causing toxicity to patients was demonstrated.

In 1941, Abraham, Florey and team published a paper in the Lancet that reported the efficacy of penicillin in the treatment of human infections.

Florey and Heatley obtained permission to travel to the USA in July 1941 to persuade scientists, administrators and pharmaceutical companies to produce penicillin, since production of the required quantities of penicillin was severely compromised by wartime conditions in Britain.

Lax noted that a pharmaceutical company asked a technician to purchase moldy fruits and vegetables and return these to the laboratory. This technician (identified as Moldy Mary) purchased a moldy cantaloupe melon that yielded a strain of *Penicillium* mold, *Penicillium chrysogenum*, that produced particularly abundant quantities of penicillin.

Penicillin was found to have a beta-lactam ring structure. Subsequently, additional antibiotics were produced through modifications at specific sites in the beta-lactam rings.

Antibiotic Discovery Processes

In a 2014 review, Gerard Wright wrote: "The drug discovery process often involves natural products or compounds that are inspired by them and modified by medicinal chemistry".

Bacteria and fungi are sources of antibiotics and other drugs. Wright noted that natural products tend to be complex macromolecules. In his review, Wright referred to the work of David Hopwood and colleagues, who characterized genes in *Streptomyces* that produce antibiotics. This was very exciting for me, since I recalled that David Hopwood was a faculty member at the Glasgow Institute of Genetics in 1967 at the time that I worked in a laboratory there. My work was on human cells, but many of the faculty at the Institute worked on fungi and micro-organisms, and David Hopwood worked on *Streptomyces*. Inspired by Wright's reference I went in search of

David Hopwood's published work and found his book published in 2007, *Streptomyces in Nature and Medicine.*

Morphologically, the actinomycete streptomycetes have external structures similar to those of fungi. They form branching filaments under some conditions. However, they also exist as rod-like cells; under some conditions they form spores in chains and under other conditions they form single spores linked by stalks to filaments. In his early work, that included electron microscopy, Hopwood proved that *Streptomyces* was a bacterial species since its DNA is not contained in a nucleus. Another interesting discovery was that the actinomycetes, including streptomycetes, can be invaded by bacteriophage. Eukaryotic organisms including fungi cannot be attacked by bacteriophages. *Streptomyces* produce antibiotics at the sporulation phase.

Different *Streptomyces* strains produce different antibiotics. The Waksman strain *Streptomyces griseus* produces streptomycin, the first antibiotic found to be active against the Tubercle bacillus.

Hopwood listed antibiotics produced by *Streptomyces* species. They include Streptomycin, Actinomycin, Streptothricin, Erythromycin, Tetracycline, Chlortetracycline, Chloramphenicol, Gentamycin, Neomycin, Nystatin, Kanamycin and Lincomycin (Clindamycin).

15 Antibiotic Resistance Mechanisms

Blair *et al.* (2015) reviewed mechanisms of antibiotic resistance. In the introduction to their review they noted that each year approximately 24,000 people in Europe die as a result of multi-drug resistant infections. In the USA, approximately 23,000 deaths per year are attributed to antibiotic resistance.

Blair *et al.* distinguished between intrinsic mechanisms of bacterial resistance to antibiotics and acquired resistance. Bacteria may be intrinsically resistant to antibiotics because antibiotics cannot cross the bacterial cell membrane, based on the composition of the cell wall. Another intrinsic resistance mechanism has to do with the existence of effective efflux pumps that rapidly eliminate antibiotics from the bacterial cell before they can impact antibiotic functions or gene expression.

Acquired resistance of bacteria to antibiotics may result through mutation in bacterial DNA or lateral transfer of genes into bacteria (through transformation, plasmid or phage) that introduce new properties into bacteria. Such property changes include alterations in properties of bacterial cell membranes, or increased efficiency in eliminating, inactivating or modifying antibiotics. Mutations may result in changes to antibiotic targets in bacteria. An example of target alteration is the acquisition of new methylase enzymes that methylate ribosomal RNA and alter the ability of antibiotics to bind to bacterial ribosomes. Polymyxin antibiotics (e.g. colistin) exert their antibacterial effect by binding to lipopolysaccharides in the bacterial cell membrane. Blair *et al.* reported that some bacteria become resistant to polymyxin antibiotics by overproducing lipopolysaccharides.

An early example of antibiotic resistance to penicillin and other beta-lactam antibiotics was the increased production of the enzyme lactamase. To overcome this resistance, beta-lactamase inhibitors were added to antibiotics.

Genomes, Mobilomes, Information Transfer — Another Mechanism of Antibiotic Resistance Acquisition

Our microbiology professor, J.N. Coetzee, was particularly interested in bacteriophage and how phage infection of bacteria altered bacterial characteristics. Doctor C.N. Crocker, a lecturer in the Microbiology Department taught us laboratory techniques. She was particularly interested in the *Salmonella typhimurium* bacteria and how different strains arose in part through transfer of material from one strain to another.

Following graduation from medical school and hospital internships than I began to concentrate on Genetics. In genetics lectures there is intense concentration on transfer of genes, but the concentration was different than during my medical school years; emphasis then was placed on how transfer first revealed that the genetic material was DNA and not protein.

Frederick Griffith in England reported in 1928 that the rough strain of *pneumococcus* bacteria was not disease causing, but that the smooth strain was highly virulent due to the presence on the smooth strain of a polysaccharide capsule. Griffith reported that, when killed S strain pneumococci were injected into mice with live R strain, contrary to expectation the mice developed infection. He concluded that the R strain had acquired characteristics from the killed S strain. His findings were subsequently confirmed by scientists in other laboratories.

At the Rockefeller institute in New York, they subsequently carried out *in vitro* experiments and demonstrated that transfer occurred between killed S strain and R strain pneumococci. In 1944, in the journal of Experimental Medicine Avery, McLeod and McCarty reported that a specific purified fraction from Smooth *pneumococcus* was responsible for transformation of R pneumococci and that the purified transforming factor was composed of desoxyribonucleic acid (now most commonly known as deoxyribonucleic acid, DNA). They noted further that following transformation the newly acquired characteristic was transmitted to subsequent generations. In their discussion the authors noted that "the primary factor which controls the occurrence and specificity of capsular development was reduplicated".

In 2007, David Hopwood noted that transformation in *pneumococcus* involved naked DNA from the S strain and a special transfer process. Introduced DNA was taken up into the host R chromosome.

Ochman *et al.* (2000) reported that the significance of lateral gene transfer was re-emphasized in the 1950s when antibiotic resistance emerged. Joshua Lederberg and colleagues investigated antibiotic sensitivity. They determined that transduction could take place through bacteriophages, viral-like particles composed of DNA and protein. Lysogenic phages led to bursting of *Salmonella* bacteria. However, not all bacteriophages were lysogenic. Lederberg and colleagues also discovered extra-chromosomal ring shaped structures in bacteria, defined as plasmids. Plasmids contained nucleic acids and were able to replicate independently of bacteria.

Salmonella enterica Variants and Plasmids

Jacobsen *et al.* (2011) reported that *Salmonella enterica* has four subspecies and each subspecies has a large number of variants referred to as serovars. Jacobsen compared DNA sequences of 35 different serovars and determined that any strain of *Salmonella* has a large stable genome and an abundance of accessory genes. The accessory genes include phage and plasmid DNA and DNA transposable elements.

Mebrhatu *et al.* (2014) reported that the accessory DNA elements in a particular *Salmonella enterica* strain are derived through lateral transfer from other strains. The smaller laterally transferred insertion sequences, these genetic elements are 0.2 to 1.5 kilobases in size. Transposons are larger than insertion sequences and they contain transposase encoding genes. In addition, they may contain antibiotic resistance genes. Integrons are laterally transferred elements that include integrase genes. Transposases and integrases promote integration of DNA into the bacterial chromosome.

Mebrhatu noted that plasmids in *Salmonella* are extra-chromosomal elements that replicate independently. Plasmids can also contain antibiotic resistance. They may also contain genes that help the host bacterial cells survive in particular environments. Phages and prophages are virus-like entities. Specific phages can transfer virulence genes.

Salmonella bacteria also acquire particular DNA segments, defined as pathogenicity islands, that may be integrated into the host chromosome; they may have lost mobility or they may retain mobility. Mebrhatu *et al.* noted that these islands are often large, 25–39 kb in length. The pathogenicity islands often include regulatory genes.

Mebrhatu *et al.* emphasized that external genetic elements transferred into bacteria need to overcome host defensive mechanisms. These include methyltransferase that cause the incoming DNA to be more susceptible to digestion by bacterial restriction endonuclease. The methylation processes and subsequent endonuclease digestion processes are referred to as modification systems.

A bacterial defense mechanism that has recently been used in biotechnology is the Crispr CAS system (Doudna and Charpentier, 2014). The system includes 24–47 bases of repeats in the bacterial chromosome DNA separated by a spacer of 20–72 nucleotides. Incorporation of invading DNA between the repeats triggers expression of a promoter upstream of the repeats and transcription of the locus that includes the invading DNA repeat. The RNA in this transcript is bound by proteins encoded by the bacterial CAS locus and this binding blocks translation of the transcript. In addition, a specific histone produced by bacteria may block expression of the inserted genes by binding to the upstream promoter region and preventing recruitment of RNA polymerase and thereby blocking transcription. The inserted genes may become non-functional pseudo genes in the bacteria. There is evidence that they are often eliminated from bacteria by deletion.

Laterally transmitted DNA may, however, in some cases become domesticated in bacteria and introduce new functions to the bacteria.

Drug Resistant *Mycobacterium tuberculosis*

A WHO fact sheet "Antimicrobial resistance" revealed that worldwide 3.6% of new cases and 20.2 % of previously treated TB cases are due to multi-drug resistant *M. tuberculosis* strains (MDR TB). MDR TB is defined as TB that is resistant to isoniazid and rifampicin. Brigden *et al.* at Medicin sans Frontiers (2015) reviewed new developments in the treatments of drug resistant tuberculosis. They noted that up to 30% of MDR cases are also resistant to injectable second-line anti-TB agents. These cases are defined as extensively drug resistant TB (XDRTB).

The WHO lists the following as first-line anti-tuberculosis drugs: ethambutol, isoniazid, pyrazinamide, rifampicin, streptomycin.

Second-line anti-tuberculosis drugs include aminoglycosides (e.g. kanamycin); polypeptide antibiotics (e.g. capreomycin, viomycin and enviomycin); fluoroquinolones (e.g. ciprofloxacin and levofloxacin); and thioamides (e.g. cycloserine and terizidone).

Reports revealed that capreomycin is derived from *Streptomyces capreolus*. Viomycin is derived from *Streptomyces puniceus*. Thioamide antibiotics, such as thioviridamide, are synthesized from nitriles.

In the Brigden *et al.* paper, the authors report that in the cohorts they studied in France, only 2% of patients with MDR TB were HIV positive, while in South Africa the HIV co-infection rate in the TB cohort they studied was 59.3%. In Armenia, HIV co-infection occurred in 4% of individuals in their cohort.

Brigden *et al.* reported encouraging results using new medications developed for treatment of tuberculosis, Bedaquiline (developed by Janssen Company in Belgium) and Delamanid (developed by Otsuka Pharmaceuticals in Japan). In addition, they noted that there is evidence that repurposed drugs including clofazamine and linezolid. However, they noted that the repurposed drugs have side effects.

The clinical trial protocols in their studies of MDR TB patients included treatment using the five recommended TB treatment drugs in both test cases and controls; in addition, Bedaquiline was added in test cases. They determined culture conversion e.g. generation of TB negative cultures following treatment. Conversion to sputum negative for TB organisms was achieved in 97% of cases in the cohort in France and 77% of cases in South Africa. In South African patients with TB and HIV positive status, antiretroviral medications were also prescribed.

It is important to note that there are also reports that HIV develops resistance to anti-retroviral drugs (Tang and Shafer, 2012).

16 Genomics and Natural Product Discovery

Jensen *et al.* (2014) reviewed aspects of genomic-based natural product research. They emphasized that genomic sequencing provides a means to assess the biosynthetic potential of micro-organism strains. These assessments include possibilities of strains to produce specific compounds, e.g. polyketides and terpenes. Jensen et al. noted that bioinformatics expertise and lack of information on pathways has hampered progress. They noted further that highly repetitive sequence motifs occur in association with biosynthetic genes and that these impair sequence assembly. They noted further that even when sequencing reveals that specific genes are present that potentially encode enzymes in specific biochemical pathways, the products of these enzymes are not always present or are not identified.

Nett *et al.* (2009) reported that genomic studies indicate many more potential biochemical pathways in bacteria than would be predicted based on the number of products identified.

The works of Jensen *et al.* and of Hopwood and colleagues have revealed that many biosynthetic pathways in bacteria are apparently silent. They noted that this might be due to culture conditions; alternatively, the apparent silence may be dependent on inadequacy of detection methods.

Jensen noted that microorganisms produce very small quantities of specific products.

Genomic-based studies that identified particular targets in bacteria that could be inhibited by specific compounds have largely failed. This may be in part due to the fact that bacteria have redundant related systems for producing key enzymes and proteins. In addition, many inhibitors of bacterial enzymes are not able to cross the bacterial cell envelope. Furthermore, a number of bacteria have efficient efflux pumps, components that are particularly efficient at removing drugs from the bacteria. This is particularly the case with gram negative organisms (Chopra, 2013).

Additional Methods for Discovery of New Antibiotics

Chopra (2013) reviewed possibilities for discovery of new antibacterial drugs in the 21st century. He noted that whole cell screening was still a major method to identify antibiotic effects. Structural-based studies were also carried out to identify small molecules that bound to targets.

Another avenue of discovery is to utilize ancillary mechanisms to facilitate uptake of antibiotics into bacterial cells. One approach is to utilize the so-called Trojan horse approach. In this approach antibacterial compounds are linked to siderophores, structures naturally involved in the uptake of iron into bacteria.

New Methods to Identify "Unculturable" Soil Microbes

An important approach to discovery of new antibiotics depends on improved capabilities to grow and screen soil microbes.

Ling et al. (2015) reported that uncultured bacteria make up 99% of all species in external environments. They developed new methods to grow and characterize soil bacteria that cannot be grown under normal culture conditions. One novel method involves use of the ichip, a multi-channel device developed by Nichols et al. (2010).

The soil sample is diluted so that approximately one bacteria per well can be pipetted into each well of the ichip. The ichip is then covered with semi-permeable membranes and the device is put back into the soil. Ling et al. reported that organisms grew in 50% of the wells and growth was facilitated by the fact that the organisms were in a favorable environment. The organisms were then screened for ability to destroy specific bacteria. In addition, genomic sequencing was carried out.

One organism derived through this approach was an *Aquabacteria*, *Eleftheria terrae*. Fractions of this organisms were purified and a specific compound was derived, Teixobactin, and its structure was determined.

Ling *et al.* reported that Teixobactin is active against *Clostridium difficile*, *Bacillus anthracis* and methicillin resistant *Staphylococcus aureus* (MRSA). Teixobactin was also active against *Mycobacterium tuberculosis*. Teixobactin is a peptidoglycan synthesis inhibitor.

Ling *et al.* reported that no toxicity was demonstrated against cultured mammalian cells. Furthermore, they determined that the compound remained active in the presence of serum. Animal efficacy studies were carried out in mice that had prior peritoneal injection with MRSA *Staphylococcus aureus*. Teixobactin proved effective in reducing infection. It was also effective in eliminating infective thigh abscess.

17 The Human Microbiome

The Human Microbiome Project was designed to characterize the microbiome at different sites in the body and to determine the microbiome status in health and disease. Initial studies involved analyses of the body sites in 300 healthy individuals. In a review of initial results, Ding and Schloss (2014) reported that microorganism taxonomies of the mouth and gut were different but related. They also reported that the microbiome showed considerable intra- and inter-personal variations. They also reported that the male and female microbiomes differed. The gut microbiome enterotypes were found to differ dependent on the content of fat and carbohydrate in the diet. Clear differences were demonstrated in the microbiome of breast fed infants and non-breast fed infants.

With respect to the microbiome in diseases, Ding and Schloss reported that gut microbiome enterotypes differed in cases of Crohn's disease and inflammatory bowel disease. The skin microbiome in individuals with psoriasis differed from that in healthy individuals.

Schloss (2009) described open source software for description and comparison of microbiome communities.

The Gut Microbiome Kwashiorkor Connection

New studies reveal that there are likely links between the altered microbiome and manifestations of Kwashiorkor. As a medical student working in pediatric clinics in South Africa we frequently encountered young children with Kwashiorkor, a form of protein energy malnutrition. These children manifested growth retardation, their arms were thin, skin abnormalities including peeling and depigmentation, their legs were often swollen and bellies were protuberant and swollen.

Kwashiorkor differs from marasmus. Both are protein energy deficiency syndromes; however, Kwashiorkor differs in that it is characterized by edema and protuberant bellies. Recent studies reveal that in marasmus protein and carbohydrates are equally deficient in the diet, while in Kwashiorkor protein deficiency is more marked than carbohydrate deficiency. Recent studies by Smith *et al.* (2013) revealed differences in the microbiome in twins with and without kwashiorkor. They transplanted stool samples from children of both groups into the guts of mice. Subsequent metabolic studies of the urine of these mice revealed that the Kwashiorkor samples led to production of abnormal metabolites. Some of these metabolites inhibited enzymes in the tricarboxylic acid metabolic cycle.

There is also evidence that antibiotic treatment reduces some of the manifestations of Kwashiorkor; ensuring adequate protein in the diet is essential of course for return to health and normal development.

Antibiotics Impact Gut Microbiome and *Clostridium difficile* Infections

During 2015, a colleague of mine sustained a relatively minor injury that led to a short hospitalization and multiple outpatient visits. He subsequently developed a *Clostridium difficile* infection that led to pseudomembranous colitis and to his death. *C. difficile* infections are an escalating problem in hospital settings, in out-patient settings and in nursing homes. There are reports indicating that 21% of hospital patients without diarrhea carry *C. difficile* organisms that they likely acquired in hospital. (Dubberke *et al.*, 2015).

In 2015, Theriot and Young reviewed the human gastro-intestinal microbiome and its functions in *C difficile* infections. They emphasized the importance of healthy microbial communities in maintenance of gut health. Nucleic acid sequencing has revealed that gut microbiota comprises between 15,000 and 36,000 different species of bacteria. Two dominant phyla include Firmicutes and Bacteroidetes. Other phyla that predominate include Proteobacteria, Actinobacteria, Verrucomicrobia and Cyanobacteria. Benefits of the gut microbiota include the breakdown of indigestible material. In addition, they generate metabolites, including short chain fatty acids and break down products of bile acids that are important for gut health. There is evidence that a five-day course of antibiotics e.g.

amoxicillin and clavulanic acid reduces the species of gut microbiota that are necessary for colonic health.

Theriot and Young reviewed the history of *C difficile*. This organism was first described in 1925 and it is a gram positive spore forming toxin producing bacillus. Antibiotics alter the composition of the intestinal microbiome and its metabolic functions, leading to the production of products that favor *C. difficile* spore germination. *Clostridium difficile* infection is reported to be frequently responsible for diarrhea in patients treated with antibiotics, and particularly those treated with broad spectrum antibiotics. Tedesco (1974) reported that 21% of patients who developed diarrhea after treatment with clindamycin subsequently developed pseudomembranous colitis. *C. difficile* was found to produce toxins Ted A and Ted B that lead to disruptions of the colon epithelium and to cell death. In patients with pseudomembranous colitis, reintroduction of organisms that constitute the healthy microbiome have proven useful in eliminating *C difficile* infections that could not be cured by antibiotics.

18 Bacterial Microfilms

Studies on bacterial microfilms have provided new information on microorganism behavior and yielded insights into infections. Biofilms form on biological and non-biological surfaces. The latter include catheters, medical devices, intubation tubes, prostheses and medical equipment. Biofilms are a particular problem in the healthcare setting. Kostakioti *et al.* (2013) reviewed aspects of biofilm generation. They noted that developmental changes occur in the organisms that form biofilms. The key developmental changes involve transformation from planktonic bacteria that float in liquid medium to bacteria that are anchored in an extra-cellular matrix that they produce. The matrix that bacteria produce protects them from host immunological processes. In addition, inter-bacterial interactions occur within the matrix and facilitate the spread of drug resistance.

Kostakioti *et al.* reported that organisms found within biofilms include *Pseudomonas aeruginosa*, *Klebsiella pneumoniae*, *Streptococcus* and *Enterococcus*.

A first step in biofilm formation involves attraction of bacteria to specific surfaces. Some bacteria, such as *Pseudomonas aeruginosa*, utilize attachment organelles to adhere to surfaces. Other bacteria secrete adhesins that facilitate binding to the eukaryotic extra-cellular matrix. One example is *Enterococcus*, that form biofilms on the endocardium and in the urinary tract.

Kostakioti *et al.* reported that adherence to surfaces leads to changes in bacterial gene expression, increased production of bacterial matrix, and to promotion of sessile protrusions that promote attachment. Furthermore, within the mature biofilm, organisms exchange products and share nutrients. As the biofilm colonies grow, organisms may be shed. Organisms in biofilms may also eventually penetrate host cell membranes and became intracellular. *Klebsiella pneumoniae* has been shown to form intra-cellular communities.

Williams *et al.* (2007) reported that there are situations where bacteria can behave cooperatively and exchange diffusible small molecules. There is also evidence that they can exchange signaling molecules that provide information on collective colony size and environmental conditions such as nutrient availability. This is referred to as quorum sensing and is based on signaling molecules that ultimately lead to changes in gene expression. One molecule related to as quorum sensing is acyl-homoserine lactone, other signaling molecules are peptides.

Tolker-Nielsen (2014) reviewed *Pseudomonas* biofilms and notes that *Pseudomonas aeruginosa* plays roles in periodontitis (gum margin infections), cystic fibrosis, urinary tract infections, mitral valve endocarditis, necrotizing fasciitis (flesh eating bacterial infection) and in medical device infections. *Pseudomonas aeruginosa* is also often involved in chronic infections such diabetes ulcers. *Pseudomonas* produces an alginate matrix.

Tolker Nielsen *et al.* noted that medical devices are often coated with platelets and host components that attract microbes. They also noted that certain virulence factors produced by biofilm bacteria kill host immune cells.

It is interesting to note that some investigators, including Lanter *et al.* (2014), have proposed that biofilms are present on arteriosclerosis plaques in blood vessels and may contribute to plaque rupture. Lanter *et al.* identified bacterial genes from *Pseudomonas* in arteriosclerosis lesions in carotid arteries.

Treatment Strategies

Kostakioti *et al.* reported that biofilm bacteria are resistant to antibiotic treatments. Resistance results in part, perhaps, because the extracellular matrix impairs diffusion of antibiotics into the bacteria. In addition, the different combinations of bacteria in close contact with each other promote transfer of antibiotic resistance genes (Donlan, 2000).

Kostakioti *et al.* noted that another strategy is to utilize anti-adhesion agents on medical devices. Such agents include nano-particles of silver and anti-microbial peptides. Another strategy is to coat medical device surfaces with enzymes that would destroy the matrix of the biofilm.

It is important to re-emphasize that biofilms form not only on syn-thetic surfaces but also on body tissues. A form of the enzyme glycoside hydrolase is used to treat cystic fibrosis patients, where biofilms form in bronchi. In cystic fibrosis, the biofilms often contain *Staphylococcus aureus*, *Pseudomonas aeruginosa* and *Hemophilus influenza*. In cystic fibrosis, in-halation of hypertonic sodium chloride 5% or 7% has proven advantageous in clearing mucus that predisposes to biofilm formation (Donaldson *et al.*, 2006). In addition, exercise proves useful.

19 Strategies to Overcome the Problem of Bacterial Antibiotic Resistance

In 2014, the World Health Organization urged countries to develop and finance plans to address the antibiotic resistance problem. In the USA, Center for Disease Control (CDC) formulated the National Strategy for Combating Antibiotic Resistant Bacteria (http://www.cdc.gov/drugresitance/threat-report-2013). There are five key goals of this strategy. The first is to reduce emergence of resistant bacteria and spread of resistant infections through more judicious use of antibiotics in healthcare systems and in the agricultural industry.

In the agricultural industry, antibiotics have been used in healthy food producing animals to promote growth. New recommendations are that use of medically important antibiotics for animal growth promotion be eliminated. The United States Department of Agriculture will undertake to develop substances that can be used as alternatives to antibiotics to promote growth.

In healthcare settings, hospitals will need to report antibiotic use. A key problem leading to inappropriate antibiotic use in healthcare settings is the inability of personal to readily distinguish between bacterial and viral infections. In addition, the lag time between acquiring samples for testing and obtaining results of the type of bacteria involved and their antibiotic sensitivities is often three days, so physicians are reduced to guessing which antibiotic to use in a specific case. The ongoing development of more efficient methods for pathogen detection and sensitivity are therefore critical. Developments of point of care diagnostic methods are particularly important particularly in rural areas. Point of care diagnostics are often based on specific proteins or DNA characteristics of a microorganism. Therefore, ongoing research efforts to identify proteins and mutant DNA sequences of resistant organisms are required and databases with relevant information must be established. The CDC report also emphasized that policies should be introduced to ensure financial re-imbursement for routine use of diagnostics in clinical settings.

The CDC report also emphasized the importance of accelerating private sector investment in development of therapeutics to treat infections. The report noted that "current private sector interest in antibiotic development is limited". In addition to promoting research to develop new antibiotics there is also increasing emphasis on development of vaccines and novel therapeutics.

Novel Antibacterial Agents

Novel classes of anti-infective substances being investigated include antimicrobial peptides produced by plants, insects, humans and even by bacteria. Steckbeck *et al.* (2014) reported that many antimicrobial peptides cause bacterial membrane rupture; they may also infiltrate bacteria and impair intra-cellular bacterial targets.

In addition to natural anti-microbial peptides, production of synthetic antimicrobial peptides is also underway. Steckbeck *et al.* reported that a specific antimicrobial peptide sometimes has activity toward several different bacteria. In addition, specific antimicrobial peptides have anti-viral properties.

Inhibitors of the bacterial enzyme type II fatty acid synthase are also being investigated as anti-infection therapeutics. Yao *et al.* (2016) reported that many bacteria cannot bypass inhibition of fatty acid synthesis. They reported that a broad spectrum of Gram positive and Gram negative organisms are eliminated by these inhibitors.

However, new therapeutics that function in elimination of bacteria *in vitro* need to go through several phases of pre-clinical and clinical trials to demonstrate absence of toxicity to humans and to prove *in vivo* effectiveness.

Investigations Into Use of Bacteriophage to Fight Bacterial Infections

Bacteriophages invade bacteria, and lytic phages can destroy bacteria. In Eastern Europe, bacteriophages have been used to treat bacterial infections for a number of years. Bacteriophages do not invade eukaryotic cells so human cells are not damaged directly by phage. However, bacteriophages have not been used to treat human infections in Western countries. Reardon (2015) reported that Western countries, including European countries and the USA, are carrying out research to determine the efficacy and safety of the use of bacteriophages to treat antibiotic resistant bacterial infections.

20 Point of Care Diagnostics

Reliable of point of care diagnostic assays that facilitate diagnosis of the microorganisms responsible for disease in a specific patient and that provide information on the antibiotic sensitivity of the responsible organism are urgently needed.

A number of point of care diagnostic techniques that are currently in use are based on analysis of specific proteins (antigens) produced by specific organisms. Other tests are based on the nucleic acid characteristic of organisms (DNA or RNA sequence). In some cases, specific nucleic acid mutations that lead to antibiotic resistance are also analyzed. One avenue of analysis involves utilization of nucleic acid amplification techniques (NAAT).

Zumla *et al.* (2014) reported that few validated point of care diagnostics were available for diagnosis of respiratory infections with the exception of the GeneXpert assay for *Mycobacterium tuberculosis* organisms and resistance to the antibiotic rifampicin. They emphasized the need for rapid diagnosis of emerging viral-caused respiratory infections. Examples of the latter include SARS (severe, acute respiratory syndrome) due to corona virus and MERS (Middle East respiratory system) corona virus.

Zumla *et al.* noted that an ideal point of care diagnostic system included kits that integrate sample preparation (e.g. extraction of nucleic acids from body fluids or cells) and pathogen detection; in addition, there should be unambiguous readout of results.

Currently available point of care diagnostic systems are based on detection of a single pathogen. However, in some situations the ability to detect multiple pathogens will be advantageous. Furthermore, in specific cases, detection of antibiotic resistance is critically important. In addition, in specific rural areas power supplies are an issue and equipment that utilizes rechargeable batteries is an advantage.

Zumla *et al.* noted that Medicine as a science involved the introduction of microscopy to identify organisms and introduction of methods to culture organisms. They noted that since the 1980s, advances in immunology and molecular genetics have added new dimensions to the science of diagnosis. These dimensions involved the use of antibodies and methodologies to examine nucleic acids. Nucleic acids can be amplified in polymerase chain reaction. These assays can be multiplexes to identify several different organisms. Molecular PCR assays were developed to rapidly detect MERS infection.

Zumla *et al.* emphasized that, although culture of organisms and identification of the organism that leads to disease in a specific patient may be the gold standard, in many cases there are specific delays in diagnosis due to the length of culture time and there are further delays in defining antibiotic sensitivity of the specific organisms. In some situations, nucleic acid sequencing offers a diagnostic method. However, sequencing of an organism directly from infected clinical material is often difficult.

Zumla *et al.* emphasized that there are differences between cases, in some cases colonization by an organism occurs. In other cases, that organism is responsible for infection. They noted that further research is required that is directed toward identification of specific factors that promote or minimize virulence. These factors likely include expression of specific genes within the organism.

There are also movements to extend point of care testing more broadly and beyond the healthcare setting. In the USA, for example, specific over-the-counter HIV tests have been approved by the FDA.

21 Defining Biomarkers to Help Distinguish Viral Diseases from Bacterial Diseases

There are ongoing efforts to develop tests that measure biomarkers in patients that help to distinguish viral infections from bacterial infection. The hope is that such tests will avoid the inappropriate use of antibiotics in patients with viral diseases. One such test involves measurement of the protein procalcitonin (PCT). Pfister *et al.* (2014) reported that procalcitonin is a reasonably accurate marker for detection of bacterial pneumonia in critically ill patients. Tsalik *et al.* (2016) reported that that presence of raised levels of procalcitonin in blood was 78% accurate in predicting bacterial infections in the acute care setting. These investigators developed a test that measured a panel of biomarkers based on altered host gene expression that achieved 87% accuracy in distinguishing between bacterial and viral infections.

22 Vaccines in the 21st Century

In the 21st century, there is marked rejuvenation of vaccine research and evidence of increased vaccine use. These changes are simulated in part by the increasing frequency of microorganism resistance to antibiotics and in part by the increasing burden of viral diseases against which effective antibiotics have not been developed.

The WHO formulated a vision for a Vaccine Action Plan, 2011 to 2020. This plan partly coincided with and built on the Global Immunization Vision and strategy for 2006 to 2020. These plans were built on consultation with 140 countries and 290 organizations. Central to these plans are the United Nations and WHO concepts that "immunization is and should be recognized as a core component of the human right to health" and that "immunization is an individual, community and governmental responsibility".

The WHO Global Vaccine action plan is based partly on the premise that the 20th century was the century of treatment that stemmed from antibiotic use to control infectious disease, while the 21st century will be a century of prevention with potential to control occurrence of debilitating infectious disease. Prevention of infectious diseases is, of course, dependent not only on the use of vaccines but also on improved sanitation, access to clean water and education.

In a 2013 publication, the WHO reported that approved vaccines were available to prevent 25 microorganism related diseases, these are listed alphabetically below:

Anthrax, Cholera, Diphtheria, Hemophilus influenza B, Hepatitis A, Hepatitis B, Hepatitis E, Human papilloma virus associated malignancies, Influenza, Japanese encephalitis, Measles, Mumps, Pertussis (whooping cough), Pneumococcal diseases, Poliomyelitis, Rabies, Rotavirus gastro-enteritis,

Tetanus, Tuberculosis, Typhoid fever, Tick-borne encephalitis, Varicella and Herpes zoster (Chicken-pox and Shingles), Yellow fever.

However, use of vaccines in low and middle income countries was often low and use in rural areas was often limited. Furthermore, production of safe vaccines is frequently insufficient. Problems also exist in vaccine procurement and delivery. In addition, further innovations are required to improve vaccine thermostability. It is also important to develop easier routes of administration, for example vaccine delivery that is not dependent on the use of syringes.

The 2013 WHO report emphasized the importance of ongoing research towards developing a vaccine that shows at least 75% efficacy against Tuberculosis, and HIV/AIDS. In addition, other microorganisms and related diseases in need of vaccine development include Cytomegalovirus, Dengue virus, hookworm, *Leishmania* and respiratory syncytial virus.

The WHO emphasized that although immunization requires funding, it also has economic returns. These could include reduction of hospitalizations and associated expenses, and improved population productivity. Education of the public on the value of vaccination is critical.

Examples of Active Vaccine Research and Development of Candidate Vaccines in 2016

Dengue fever

Collaboration between the USA National Institutes of Health (NIH) and the Butantan Institute in Brazil has led to production of a vaccine against Dengue fever. In January 2016, this vaccine was reported to be in multi-center Phase 2 clinical trials. The news release reported that over 400 million cases of Dengue fever occur in the tropics and sub-tropics (https://www.niaid.nih.gov/diseases-conditions/dengue-fever). Four different sub-types of dengue virus are transmitted by the mosquito *Aedes aegypti*.

Polio

I remember clearly the polio epidemics that occurred in South Africa in the late 1940s and early 1950s. I also remember the press photographs of people encased in iron lungs, with only their heads emerging. The iron lung was used to maintain breathing following paralysis of muscles that controlled breathing. I also have memories of friends and colleagues who had recovered from polio but who had residual paralysis of lower limbs. The development of the polio vaccine and its availability by the late 1950s seemed like a miracle.

Emerging Problems with use of Attenuated Virus Vaccines

The polio vaccine developed by Salk contained inactivated (killed) polio virus and is administered by injection. The polio vaccine developed by Sabin contained an attenuated (weakened) form of live polio virus and is administered orally (Oshinsky, 2005).

Several doses of the oral vaccine are required to induce adequate immunity. A single dose of the oral vaccine is most often insufficient to induce adequate immunity. In addition, in situations where an individual is unable to mount an adequate immune response, the virus in the oral polio vaccine persists in the gastro-intestinal tract of the vaccine recipient and can accumulate in the environment. In addition, the persisting attenuated virus can undergo mutation and give rise to genetically divergent neurotropic viruses referred to as vaccine derived poliovirus (VDPV). This is also referred to as circulating vaccine derived polio virus, cVDPV. In 2015, Diop et al. and the CDC USA Center for Disease control) reported that polio cases due to indigenous emergent cVDPV had occurred in Pakistan, Nigeria, Madagascar and South Sudan. In addition, genetically variant VDPV was imported into Cameroon, Kenya and Niger. There were also reports that genetically variant forms of VDPD were identified in sewage in Brazil, China, Israel and Nigeria.

The WHO reported (2015) that poliomyelitis due to wildtype poliovirus was reported in a patient from Syria. Wildtype poliovirus also exists in Pakistan and Afghanistan.

The decreased immune response in cases of immunodeficiency such as occurs in HIV/AIDS makes use of oral attenuated polio vaccine a particular problem. The WHO recommended changes in the types of oral polio vaccine. They also instructed that oral vaccine be used after one dose of injectable inactivated polio vaccine.

Possibilities for Development of Effective HIV Vaccines

The high frequency of mutations in many of the genes in the HIV virus constitutes one impediment to development of effective HIV vaccines. Another problem is the inability of the host system to mount an effective immune defense.

Some patients do, however, develop antibodies that cross-react with the HIV virus. Zhou et al. (2010) determined that in some patients with HIV/ AIDS, neutralizing antibodies developed against a specific component of the HIV envelope, a glycoprotein designated gp120. This glycoprotein binds to the human T lymphocyte receptor CD4.

Zhou (2010) isolated specific gp120 producing B cells from a patient who produced these antibodies. They derived a cell line that could be cultured long-term and that continued to produce anti-gp120 antibodies. This antibody, designated VRCO1, has subsequently been shown to re- duce circulating HIV virus in volunteers with HIV/AIDS. These circulating antibodies do not, however, impact viruses that are present in cells.

VRCO1 antibody therapy may be an option in treatment of early onset HIV/AIDS infection (Lynch et al., 2015). More importantly, studies of the actions of the interactions of the VRCO1 antibody and HIV virus provide insight into HIV targets for vaccines. In addition, important insights have been obtained into mechanisms through which HIV binds to T lymphocytes and enters these cells.

Cohen (2015) reported that researchers have demonstrated that the gp120 envelope protein of HIV binds to the CD4 receptor on T lymphocytes. This binding leads to a conformational change in the virus that exposed another HIV protein that binds to a second T lymphocyte receptor, CCR5. Both of these T cell binding functions are necessary for HIV to enter into T lymphocytes. Antibodies against gp120 protein inhibit the first phase of HIV binding to T lymphocytes. In 2015, a vaccine that generates antibodies to gp120 is being investigated (Excler et al., 2015).

Vaccine Development

Barocchi and Rappuoli (2015) reviewed traditional types of vaccines and new approaches to vaccine development. Traditionally, three types of vaccines were used to immunize against pathogens. The first type contained organisms killed by heat or chemicals. The second type contained live organisms. These vaccines included organisms that had been weakened (attenuated) through multiple passages in *in vitro* culture. In some cases, the live organism in vaccines were non-pathogenic organisms that were antigenically closely related to the pathogenic organism. The third type of traditional vaccines includes toxoid vaccines, where a specifically damaging product produced by the organism was inactivated and used to stimulate production of antibodies in the host. An example of a toxoid vaccine is the Diphtheria vaccine.

Barocchi and Rappuoli reported that subunit vaccines are increasingly being developed. In these vaccines a particular fragment of the organism, often a surface protein, is used to produce a vaccine. In some cases, a specific component of the organism, for example the polysaccharide component of the outer membrane is complexed (conjugated) *in vitro* to specific proteins known to be highly immunogenic. The conjugate serves as a vaccine to elicit an antibody response in the host.

Other newer vaccines include genomic material from microorganisms. Next generation sequencing and molecular technologies facilitate isolation of specific important genes from microorganisms. In some cases, the genes are cloned into replicating viruses to produce modified vaccines.

Economic Factors in Vaccine Development

Provision of existing vaccines to developing countries has been greatly facilitated by the Global Alliance for Vaccines and Immunization (GAVI), The Vaccine Fund and the Bill and Melinda Gates Foundation. However, Barocchi and Rappuoli (2015) reported that significant difficulties remain in developing countries due to the shortage of vaccines required by those countries but not required by the Western World. They noted that this difficulty stems from the lack of financial incentives for the private sector.

Barocchi and Rappuoli reported that several institutions were recently established to expedite design and production of vaccines for use in developing countries. Examples of such institutes include the Novartis Vaccine Institute in Italy and the Vaccine Institute in Korea. Other institutes dedicated to vaccine development include public–private partnerships such as the Glaxo-Smith-Kline NIH partnership and Sanofi Pasteur Institute. A lead project of the Novartis Vaccine Institute is the development of vaccines for typhoid fever, caused by *Salmonella enterica*.

Vaccines against Ebola

The Ebola epidemic that occurred in West Africa in 2014 led to the deaths of many thousands of people. International consortia were formed to develop vaccines and plans evolved to expedite clinical trials of newly developed vaccines. Tully et al. (2015) reported information on the development of two candidate Ebola vaccines and on innovative clinical trials.

Studies on the Ebola virus revealed that a specific glycoprotein on the surface of that virus stimulated immunity and was a target for vaccine development. Through molecular technologies this Ebola glycoprotein was moved to and expressed in a simian adenovirus (CAD3) to develop the CAD3-EBOV vaccine. The key Ebola virus glycoprotein was also moved to and expressed in a recombinant vesicular stomatitis virus to develop the rVSV-EBOV vaccine. These vaccines passed safety tests. New clinical trial procedures were designed to expedite delivery of these vaccines to individuals at risk.

It is interesting to note that funding for the development and clinical trials of the rVSV-EBOV vaccine came from the WHO, The Wellcome trust, Medicin sans Frontieres, the Norwegian government and the Canadian government.

Henao-Restrepo et al. (2015) reported results of a ring vaccination cluster randomized trial carried out in New Guinea using the rVSV-EBOV vaccine. In these trials, confirmation of a new case of Ebola, contacts of the case and contacts of the primary contacts were recruited to the clinical trial. These recruits include persons 18 years or older who were not pregnant and not breast feeding. Two groups were set-up; in the first group (4,123 people) immediate vaccination of the contact occurred. In the second group (3,528 individuals) vaccination occurred after 10 days or more. This trial was carried out from April to July. In the immediate vaccination cluster, no cases of Ebola developed. In the delayed vaccination group, 16 cases of Ebola occurred. One case of serious vaccine effect occurred, this was a febrile episode that resolved.

Henao-Restrepo et al. (2015) reported that the rVSV-EBOV vaccine was likely highly efficacious and safe in preventing EBOLA infections.

23 New Economic Approaches to Financing New Medications

Barocchi and Rappuoli (2015) discussed new approaches and models to fund development of vaccines and other medications needed in low income countries. The Advance Market Commitment (AMC) established by the Global Vaccine Action Plan (GAVI) promoted donors to subsidize the costs of vaccines that are needed in developing countries. AMC also functions in promoting suppliers to make funds available for research development and staff training.

Another important interesting proposed new funding mechanism is the Health Impact Fund (HIF). The HIF plan incentivizes companies making new medications to register with the HIF. The companies would then make drugs available at cost to sites where they were needed. They would subsequently be reimbursed by the HIF based on the impact of the medicine on solving a specific problem.

The HIF proposal as outlined by Banerjee et al. (2010) grew out of observations that market forces and intellectual property rights provided little incentive for innovations in finding cures for diseases prevalent in low income countries.

An example of progress toward goals similar to those of the HIF proposal was the pledge in 2009 by the global chief executive of Glaxo Smith Kline (GSK) to reduce prices of GSK patented drugs in developing countries and to invest in the local healthcare structures in those countries. In addition, he proposed a plan to share profits from GSK patents and intellectual property income. Needless to say, these philanthropic measures were questioned by critics.

Questions of patent rights and their relationship to price mark-ups are constantly being discussed and current practices have both supporters and critics.

Cohen (in a feature article in Science magazine in 2016) reported that newly developed vaccines against a number of important diseases are languishing in freezers. These include potentially useful vaccines that have been proven effective in animal studies and in some cases even in small studies in humans. However, funds were not available for additional comprehensive testing. Examples of vaccines in this in limbo state include vaccines against Marburg virus, Ebola Sudan, Rift valley fever, Chikungunya, West Nile virus, Middle Eastern respiratory virus MERS, South–Asian Respiratory virus (SARS) and a vaccine against hookworm.

References

Abraham EP, Chain E, Fletchér CM, *et al.* (1941). Further observations on penicillin. *Lancet* **238(6155):**177–189.

Avery OT, Macleod CM, McCarty M. (1944). Studies on the chemical nature of the substance inducing transformation of pneumococcal types: induction of transformation by a desoxyribonucleic acid fraction isolated from Pneumococcus Type III. *J Exp Med* **79(2):**137–58. PMID:19871359.

Banerjee A, Hollis A, Pogge T. (2010). The Health Impact Fund: incentives for improving access to medicines. *Lancet* **9**: 375(9709):166-9. doi:10.1016/S0140-6736(09)61296-4. PMID:20109894.

Barocchi MA, Rappuoli R. (2015). Delivering vaccines to the people who need them most. *Philos Trans R Soc Lond B Biol Sci* **370(1671):** pii: 20140150. doi: 10.1098/rstb.2014.0150. PMID:25964460.

Blair JM, Webber MA, Baylay AJ, *et al.* (2015). Molecular mechanisms of antibiotic resistance. *Nat Rev Microbiol* **13(1):**42–51. doi: 10.1038/nrmicro3380. PMID:25435309.

Brigden G, Hewison C, Varaine F. (2015). New developments in the treatment of drug-resistant tuberculosis: clinical utility of bedaquiline and delamanid. *Infect Drug Resist* **8:**367–78. doi: 10.2147/IDR.S68351. eCollection 2015. PMID:26586956.

Brown ED, Wright GD. (2016). Antibacterial drug discovery in the resistance era. *Nature* **529(7586):**336–43. doi: 10.1038/nature17042. PMID:26791724.

Chain E, Florey HW, Adelaide MB, *et al.* (1940). Penicillin as a chemotherapeutic agent. *Lancet* **236(6104):**226–28.

Chopra I. (2013). The 2012 Garrod lecture: discovery of antibacterial drugs in the 21st century. *J Antimicrob Chemother* **68(3):**496–505. doi: 10.1093/jac/dks436. PMID:23134656.

Coates AR, Halls G, Hu Y. (2011). Novel classes of antibiotics or more of the same? *Br J Pharmacol* **163(1):**184–94. doi: 10.1111/j.1476-5381.2011.01250.x. PMID:21323894.

Cohen J. (2016). AIDS pioneer finally brings AIDS vaccine to clinic. *Science Magazine* Oct. 8, 2016. DOI: 10.1126/science.aad4697.

Dengue https://www.niaid.nih.gov/diseases-conditions/dengue-fever

Ding T, Schloss PD. (2014). Dynamics and associations of microbial community types across the human body. *Nature* **509(7500):**357–60. doi: 10.1038/nature13178. PMID:24739969.

Diop OM, Burns CC, Sutter RW, *et al.* (2015). Update on vaccine-derived polioviruses — Worldwide, January 2014–March 2015. Centers for disease control and prevention. *Morbidity and mortality weekly report* **64(23):**640–646. Online at: http://www.cdc.gov/mmwr/preview/mmwrhtml/mm6423a4.htm.

Donaldson SH, Bennett WD, Zeman KL, *et al.* (2006). Mucus clearance and lung function in cystic fibrosis with hypertonic saline. *N Engl J Med* **354(3):**241–50. PMID:16421365.

Donlan RM. (2000). Role of biofilms in antimicrobial resistance. *ASAIO J* **46(6):** S47–52. Erratum in: *ASAIO J* 2001 **47(1):**99. PMID:11110294.

Doudna JA, Charpentier E. (2014). Genome editing. The new frontier of genome engineering with CRISPR-Cas9. *Science* **346(6213):**1258096. doi: 10.1126. PMID:25430774.

Dubberke ER, Reske KA, Seiler S, *et al.* (2015). Risk factors for acquisition and loss of *Clostridium difficile* colonization in hospitalized patients. *Antimicrob Agents Chemother* **59(8):** 4533-43. doi: 10.1128/AAC.00642-15. PMID:25987626.

Excler JL, Robb ML, Kim JH. (2015). Prospects for a globally effective HIV-1 vaccine. *Am J Prev Med* **49 (6 Suppl 4):** S307-18. doi: 10.1016/j.amepre.2015.09.004. Review. PMID: 26590431.

Griffith F. (1928). The significance of pneumococcal types. *J Hyg (Lond)* **27(2):** 113–59. PMID:20474956.

Henao-Restrepo AM, Longini IM, Egger M, *et al.* (2015). Efficacy and effectiveness of an rVSV-vectored vaccine expressing Ebola surface glycoprotein: interim results from the Guinea ring vaccination cluster-randomised trial. *Lancet* **386(9996):**857–66. doi: 10.1016/S0140-6736(15)61117-5. PMID: 26248676.

Hopwood DA. (2007). *Streptomyces in Nature and Medicine.* Oxford University Press.

Jacobsen A, Hendriksen RS, Aaresturp FM, *et al.* The Salmonella enterica pan-genome. *Microb Ecol* **62(3):**487–504. doi: 10.1007/s00248-011-9880-1. PMID:21643699.

Jensen PR, Chavarria KL, Fenical W, *et al.* (2014). Challenges and triumphs to genomics-based natural product discovery. *J Ind Microbiol Biotechnol* **41(2):**203–9. doi: 10.1007/s10295-013-1353-8. PMID:24104399.

Kostakioti M, Hadjifrangiskou M, Hultgren SJ. (2013). Bacterial biofilms: development, dispersal, and therapeutic strategies in the dawn of the postantibiotic era. *Cold Spring Harb Perspect Med* **3(4):**a010306. doi: 10.1101/cshperspect. a010306. PMID: 23545571.

Kovacs DJ (2000). http://www.medscape.com/viewarticle/405773_3.

Lanter BB, Sauer K, Davies DG. (2014). Bacteria present in carotid arterial plaques are found as biofilm deposits which may contribute to enhanced risk of plaque rupture. *MBio* **5(3):**e01206–14. doi: 10.1128/mBio.01206-14. PMID:24917599.

Lax E (2004). *The mold in Dr. Florey's coat.* Henry Holt and Company.

Lederberg J, Lederberg EM. (1952). Replica plating and indirect selection of bacterial mutants. *J Bacteriol* **63(3):**399–406. PMID:14927572.

Ling LL, Schneider T, Peoples AJ, et al. (2015). A new antibiotic kills pathogens without detectable resistance. *Nature* **517(7535):**455–9. Erratum: *Nature* (2015) **520(7547):**388. doi: 10.1038/nature14098. PMID:25561178.

Lok C. (2015). Mining the microbial dark matter. *Nature* **522(7556):**270–3. doi: 10.1038/522270a. PMID:26085253.

Lynch RM, Boritz E, Coates EE et al. (2015). Virologic effects of broadly neutralizing antibody VRC01 administration during chronic HIV-1 infection. *Sci Transl Med* **7(319):**319ra206. doi: 10.1126/scitranslmed.aad5752. PMID:26702094.

Mebrhatu MT, Cenens W, Aertsen A. (2014). An overview of the domestication and impact of the Salmonella mobilome. *Crit Rev Microbiol* **40(1):**63–75. doi: 10.3109/1040841X.2012.755949. PMID:23356413.

Nett M, Ikeda H, Moore BS. (2009). Genomic basis for natural product biosynthetic diversity in the actinomycetes. *Nat Prod Rep* **26(11):**1362–84. doi: 10.1039/b817069j. PMID:19844637.

Nichols D, Cahoon N, Trakhtenberg EM, et al. (2010). Use of ichip for high-throughput *in situ* cultivation of "uncultivable" microbial species. *Appl Environ Microbiol* **76(8):**2445–50. doi: 10.1128/AEM.01754-09. PMID:20173072.

Ochman H, Lawrence JG, Groisman EA. (2000). Lateral gene transfer and the nature of bacterial innovation. *Nature* **405(6784):**299–304. PMID:10830951.

Oshinsky DM (2005). *Polio an American Story.* Oxford University Press.

Pfister R, Kochanek M, Leygeber T, et al. (2014). Procalcitonin for diagnosis of bacterial pneumonia in critically ill patients during 2009 H1N1 influenza pandemic: a prospective cohort study, systematic review and individual patient data meta-analysis. *Crit Care* **18(2):**R44. doi: 10.1186/cc13760. PMID:2461248.

Reardon S. (2015). Bacterial arms race revs up. *Nature* **521(7553):**402–3. doi: 10.1038/521402a. PMID:26017421.

Schloss PD. (2009). A high-throughput DNA sequence aligner for microbial ecology studies. *PLoS One* **4(12):**e8230. doi: 10.1371/journal.pone.0008230. PMID:20011594.

Smith MI, Yatsunenko T, Manary MJ, *et al.* (2013). Gut microbiomes of Malawian twin pairs discordant for kwashiorkor. *Science* **339(6119):**548–54. doi: 10.1126/science.1229000. PMID:23363771.

Steckbeck JD, Deslouches B, Montelaro RC. (2014). Antimicrobial peptides: new drugs for bad bugs? *Expert Opin Biol Ther* **14(1):**11–4. doi: 10.1517/14712598.2013.844227. PMID:24206062.

Tang MW, Shafer RW. (2012). HIV-1 antiretroviral resistance: scientific principles and clinical applications. *Drugs* **72(9):**e1–25. doi: 10.2165/11633.630-000000000-00000. PMID:22686620.

Tedesco FJ, Barton RW, Alpers DH. (1974). Clindamycin-associated colitis. A prospective study. *Ann Inter Med* **81(4):**429-33. PMID:4412460.

Theriot CM, Young VB. (2015). Interactions between the gastrointestinal microbiome and clostridium difficile. *Annu Rev Microbiol* **69:**445–61. doi: 10.1146/annurev-micro-091014-104115. PMID:26488281.

Tolker-Nielsen T (2014). Pseudomonas aeruginosa biofilm infections: from molecular biofilm biology to new treatment possibilities. *APMIS Suppl* **138:** 1–51. doi: 10.1111/apm.12335. PMID:25399808.

Tsalik EL, Henao R, Nichols M, *et al.* (2016). Host gene expression classifiers diagnose acute respiratory illness etiology. *Sci Transl Med* **8(322):**322ra11. doi: 10.1126/scitranslmed.aad6873. PMID: 26791949.

Tully CM, Lambe T, Gilbert SC, Hill AV. (2015) Emergency Ebola response: a new approach to the rapid design and development of vaccines against emerging diseases. *Lancet Infect Dis* **15(3):**356–9. doi: 10.1016/S1473-3099(14)71071-0. Review. Erratum in: HYPERLINK Lancet Infect Dis. 2015 Mar; 15(3):263. PMID:25595637.

Williams P, Winzer K, Chan WC, Cámara M. (2007). Look who's talking: communication and quorum sensing in the bacterial world. *Philos Trans R Soc Lond B Biol Sci* **362(1483):**1119–34. PMID:17360280.

World Health Organization WHO (2014). Summary: Global immunization coverage in 2013 www.who.int/immunization/monitoring_surveillance/global_immunization_data.pdf

World Health Organization WHO (2014). Fact sheet: Antimicrobial resistance http://www.who.int/mediacentre/factsheets/fs194/en/ (accessed on December 27th 2015).

World Health Organization WHO: Maternal and Neonatal Tetanus (MNT) elimination http://www.who.int/immunization/diseases/MNTE_initiative/en/ (accessed on Sep 7th 2015).

World Health Organization WHO: Global Vaccine action plan 2011–2020 http://www.who.int/immunization/global_vaccine_action_plan/en/

Wright G. (2014). Perspective: Synthetic biology revives antibiotics. *Nature* **509(7498):**S13. doi: 10.1038/509S13a. PMID:24784423.

Yao J, Bruhn DF, Frank MW, *et al.* (2016). Activation of Exogenous Fatty Acids to Acyl-Acyl Carrier Protein Cannot Bypass FabI Inhibition in Neisseria. *J Biol Chem* **291(1):**171–81. doi: 10.1074/jbc.M115.699462. PMID:26567338.

Zumla A, Al Tawfiq JA, Enne VI, *et al.* (2014). Rapid point of care diagnostic tests for viral and bacterial respiratory tract infections--needs, advances, and future prospects. *Lancet Infect Dis* **14(11):**1123–35. doi: 10.1016/S1473-3099(14)70827-8. PMID:25189349.

Zhou T, Georgiev I, Wu X, *et al.* (2010). Structural basis for broad and potent neutralization of HIV-1 by antibody VRC01. *Science* **329(5993):**811–7. doi: 10.1126/science.1192819. PMID:20616231.

PART V

Nuclei, Chromosomes, Genomes and Gene Products

24 Entering Genetics Through Studies on Nuclei, Chromatin and Chromosomes

My introduction to studies in genetics began when, in 1966, I undertook a research project to study sex chromatin in a series of patients. The study specifically involved studies of the so-called Barr bodies in epidermal cells in buccal smears and the study of specific appendages, known as drumsticks on polymorphonuclear white blood cells present in blood smears.

Barr bodies were shown by Graham and Barr in 1952 to be derived from the X chromosome and to be present in cells in the interphase of cell division. Ohno and Makino (1961) reported that Barr bodies were absent from cells from males, who normally have a single X chromosome. In females with two X chromosomes a single Barr body was present. Mary Lyon (1963) established that in a normal female with two X chromosomes, one X chromosome is inactivated and gives rise to the Barr body.

Davidson and Smith (1954) first reported a morphological sex difference in polymorphonuclear leukocytes. They described the sex specific body in leukocytes of females as having a head approximately 1.5 microns in diameter that was joined to the rest of the nucleus by a fine thread. They referred to this structure as a drumstick.

Ferguson-Smith (1965) reported that abnormalities in Barr body counts and Barr body size occurred in individuals with abnormalities of X chromosomes. For example, in females with Turner syndrome, Barr bodies were absent from cells and chromosome studies revealed the presence of a single X chromosome. Turner syndrome is associated with short stature and impaired ovarian function. Patients with unusually small Barr bodies were found to have deletions of the X chromosome.

In the sex chromatin research study I examined buccal smears and blood smears from 130 males and 64 females. I identified three patients with abnormal sex chromatin, and chromosome studies were subsequently undertaken on these patients.

In one female patient, I identified two sex chromatin bodies in a significant proportion of cells and chromosome studies revealed that this patient was mosaic, with two populations of cells, one with XX chromosome composition and another cell population with XXX chromosomes.

In a male patient I identified the presence of a Barr body is a significant proportion of cells and this patient was found to have an XXY karyotype and features of Klinefelter syndrome. Males with this syndrome frequently have small testes and low levels of testosterone. They may also manifest breast enlargement.

In a patient designated as male, I identified sex chromatin bodies in buccal cells and in peripheral blood leucocytes. The karyotype in this patient was 46XX. This patient had large breasts and external genitalia manifested male features; testes were not detected. Surgical studies revealed that gonads were present in the abdominal cavity in the position of ovaries and an underdeveloped uterus was present. Histological studies revealed that the right gonad had features of ovary and testis. In the left gonad, ovarian tissue was present. At that time the patient was diagnosed as a case of hermaphroditism. However, this term is no longer used. In accord with new nomenclature, the diagnosis in this patient would be 46XX disorder of sexual development.

Training in Tissue Culture and Cytogenetics

Following the studies described above, I was fortunate enough to receive further training. In Glasgow, Scotland I received training in culture of human tissues in the laboratory of Professor Guido Pontecorvo under the supervision of Dr. Joan MacNab and training in cytogenetic techniques in the laboratories of Dr. Malcom Ferguson-Smith.

The studies I carried out in Glasgow were centered around analysis of chromosomes in tissues of spontaneously aborted fetuses. Our studies and those carried out at a number of different sites in several countries revealed that chromosome abnormalities likely led to spontaneous abortion in a significant percentage of cases.

Following this training, I returned to South Africa and was able to continue chromosome studies as physicians and families searched for causative factors in children with congenital malformations and in cases of intellectual disability.

It is now appropriate to consider developments and insights gained into the pathogenesis of the conditions I initially sought to understand.

Progress in Understanding Disorders of Sexual Development

New diagnostic categories have been defined that replace older terms such as "intersex conditions" and "hermaphroditism". These terms include: 46XY disorders of sexual development (DSD), 46XX DSD, ovotesticular DSD, 46XX testicular DSD, 46XY complete gonadal dysgenesis (Ono and Harley, 2012).

Confirmation of the patient's karyotype is critical to the new classification. Ultrasound studies to investigate gonadal position and structure and position of secondary sexual organs are required in addition to histologic studies. Analyses of hormone levels and molecular studies are also beneficial.

During the past 50 years, considerable progress has been made in defining factors involved in sexual differentiation and development. Sex development has been shown to involve not only genes that map to sex chromosomes X and Y but genes that map to autosomes are also important.

Disorders of sexual development are currently defined as disorders in which development of chromosomal, gonadal or anatomical sex is atypical (Ohnesorg et al., 2014).

Though much is now known about genes and pathways involved in sexual development, questions remain.

An important breakthrough in understanding sexual development was the discovery of the SRY gene on the Y chromosome and the critical role of the product of the SRY gene in testis development. Other key factors in testis development are SOX9 and NR5A1. Sox9 deficiency leads to 46XY gonadal dysgenesis. SOX9 over-expression (e.g. due to duplication of the segment on chromosome 17q24.3 that contains the SOX9 gene) leads to 46XX testicular disorder of sexual development.

The NR5A1 gene (that maps to chromosome 9q33) encodes a transcription factor also known as a steroidogenic factor. Deficiency of this factor leads to 46XY disorder of sexual development. SRY and NR5A1 exert their effects by binding to a specific enhancer sequence within the SOX9 gene (Ostrer, 2014).

SOX9 is upregulated in Sertoli cells and SOX 9 likely induces Sertoli cell differentiation in the gonad and is key to testis differentiation. Sertoli cells also produce anti-Mullerian hormone, that leads to repression of structures that would generate oviducts. SOX9 inhibits expression of transcription factors that promote expression of the protein beta-catenin, that is particularly important in female sexual development.

In recent years, additional information has emerged regarding sex determining transcription factors and signaling molecules and their cofactors. Map kinases have been shown to play important roles. Genomic studies including microarray studies that demonstrate copy number changes in genomic segments in specific chromosomal regions have been shown to lead to abnormalities of sexual differentiation. In addition, genome sequencing studies have revealed mutations in specific signaling genes. MAP3K1 defects have been found in 13–18% of cases with 46XY gonadal dysgenesis (Ostrer, 2014). Other important signaling molecules in male sex determination include FGF9 and FGFR2.

Molecular studies in patients and studies investigating the effect of specific gene mutations in the mouse have revealed that many genes and regulatory factors play roles in sexual differentiation.

Following migration of germ cells into the gonad in the early embryo, the somatic cells of the gonad produce factors that promote differentiation of the gonad and subsequent differentiation of secondary sex organs. In the testes, Sertoli cells are key to production of SRY and SOX9 and Leydig cells produce testosterone that promotes differentiation of the Wolffian duct system. In the ovary, the support cells (granulosa cells and thecal cells) play essential roles. The thecal cells produce androstenedione and the granulosa cells produce enzymes that convert this to estrogen.

Ono and Harley (2012) documented gene regulatory networks in gonadal development based on studies in mice and humans. A series of transcription factors and their receptors regulate expression of SRY.

Ono and Harley (2012) documented specific genes involved in the differentiation of the female gonad. Signaling by beta-catenin is essential for female gonad development and this is stimulated by

RSPO1 and other genes including WNT4. Specific genes involved in the differentiation of the female gonads also repress testicular development.

In the male gonad, expression of SOX9 upregulates FGF9 and this represses WNT4 that is essential for female gonad development.

Ono and Harley documented 15 genes that have been shown to be defective in cases of 46XY DSD. They documented seven genes that have been shown to be defective in cases of 46 XX DSD.

Defects in specific hormone related genes also play roles in disorders of sexual differentiation. These include genes that produce products involved in steroid synthesis, products that encode steroid receptors (e.g. androgen receptor AR) and products involved in metabolism of steroids. In some cases, specific gene mutations lead to DSD. In other cases, specific deletions and duplications lead to DSD.

Disorders of sexual development (DSD) may occur as components of specific syndromes that include abnormalities that involve other body systems. For example, DSD occurs in cases of Bardet–Biedl syndrome. Defects in at least nine different genes lead to Bardet–Biedl syndrome

Key Genes in Male Sexual Differentiation

SRY, sex determining region Y.

SF1 (NR5A1) nuclear receptor subfamily 5 group A transcriptional activator.

SOX9 SRY box9, DNA binding protein, transcription regulator.

CBX2 chromobox 2, transcriptional repressor.

WT1 Wilms tumor 1, urogenital tract development.

MAP3K kinase involved in signaling.

AMH anti-Mullerian hormone, represses development of ducts that give rise to uterus, fallopian tubes.

FGF9 fibroblast growth factor 9.

Key Genes in Female Sexual Development

WNT4 WNT family 4 signaling molecule, antagonizes testes developing factor.

CNNTB1 Beta-catenin, regulates cell growth and adhesion.

FOXL2 Forkhead box-like, DNA binding protein plays a role in ovarian development.

ARX Aristaless homeobox, involved in development.

RSPO1 R-spondin 1, interacts with WNT4.

Abnormalities in sexual differentiation due to abnormalities in steroid hormone synthesis or function.

AR Androgen receptor.

CYP11A1, CYP11B1, CYP17A1 Cytochrome p450 enzymes involved in synthesis of cholesterol and steroids.

CYP21A2 cytochrome p450 enzyme involved in steroid synthesis, deficient in adrenal hyperplasia.

CYP17A1 Defects in this gene may also lead to adrenal hyperplasia.

CYP19A1

CYP21A

25 Excursions into Enzymes, Polymorphisms and Biochemistry

Adventures in Biochemical Genetics

When I was a graduate student in London, I carried out studies on the alcohol metabolizing enzyme alcohol dehydrogenase. The purpose of the studies was to determine the degree of genetic variation in this enzyme and to analyze expression of this enzyme during human development.

I carried out extensive studies on different forms of the enzyme alcohol dehydrogenase that were separated on gel electrophoresis and visualized through a staining procedure that used ethanol as substrate, nicotinamide adenine dinucleotide (NAD) as co-enzyme and dyes that detected the conversion of NAD to the reduced form at positons on the gel where enzyme was present.

We were able to study tissue samples from spontaneously aborted fetuses, a few samples from infants who died in early life and samples from adults. The tissue samples included liver, lung, kidney and gastro-intestinal tract. The restricted expression of certain forms (isozymes) of alcohol dehydrogenase in the different tissues allowed us to formulate a hypothesis proposing that three different gene loci determined production of the isozymes we saw on gel electrophoresis. We designated these loci as ADH1, ADH2 and ADH3. The studies on different tissues and at different gestational ages revealed that ADH1 was expressed in fetal liver from early fetal life onwards. In later fetal life, the ADH2 locus was expressed. Expression of the ADH3 gene locus in liver commenced in the neonatal period.

The ADH2 locus was expressed in lung from early fetal life onwards and continued in adult life. The ADH3 locus was expressed in intestinal tissue and in kidney from early fetal life onwards.

The analysis of ADH isozymes at different life stages provided glimpses into the wonders of the regulation of gene expression at different times and in different tissues (Smith et al., 1971, 1972).

In samples of biopsy tissue we sometimes noted an extra isozyme that had a slower electrophoretic mobility than the ADH1, ADH2 and ADH3 isozymes. This additional more anodal form seemed likely to be derived from a separate unrelated locus.

We also carried out analyses on enzyme activity, and enzyme kinetics. Through such studies and through analyses on differences in electrophoretic mobility we determined that there were individual differences (polymorphisms) in the products of the ADH2 and the ADH loci. An individual variation in the ADH2 gene product was noted in liver samples from about 10% of individuals. The ADH form turned out to also have altered enzyme kinetic properties, with more rapid production of aldehyde than the more typical product of AD2H. This form with altered kinetics corresponded to the atypical ADH described by von Wartburg and Schurch in 1964.

Testing Hypotheses on the Subunit Structure of the ADH1, ADH2 and ADH3 Gene Products

The isozyme patterns we observed in adult livers were complicated due to the fact that ADH1, ADH2 and ADH3 gene products were present and in addition there were polymorphisms in ADH2 and ADH3, so that patterns in individual samples could differ.

We hypothesized that each single polypeptide product derived from an ADH1, ADH2 or ADH3 locus could associate with a like polypeptide chain from the same locus or with a polypeptide chain from one of the other two loci.

In order to investigate the hypothesis, we purified specific isozymes and then subjected them to conditions to disassociate them, followed by conditions to re-associate sub-units. Through these experiments we were able to prove that our hypothesis on the subunit structure were confirmed (Smith et al., 1973).

Molecular Genetic Studies on Alcohol Dehydrogenase

In 1981, I joined the faculty at the University of California at Irvine and began to learn techniques in Molecular Biology. I was fortunate enough to be able to collaborate with Gregg Duester and Wes Hatfield and together we were able to isolate clones for the three genes ADH1, ADH2 and ADH3. We mapped these genes to the long arm of human chromosome 4 (Duester *et al.*, 1986).

Specific DNA sequence differences between the three different gene loci were identified; it was possible to analyze individual variations (polymorphisms) at the DNA level. Of particular interest was the fact that the "atypical" form of ADH2 that differed in its electrophoretic and kinetic properties could be readily identified through DNA studies. The ADH2 form identified as "atypical" in European populations turned out to be very common in individuals from China and Japan.

We also noted that there were activity differences between the ADH3 locus alleles ADH3-1 (gamma 1) and ADH3-2 (gamma 2).

Additional ADH Gene Loci

It is now known that 7 ADH genes map to human chromosome 4q21.1. Different nomenclatures have been proposed. The ADH1, ADH2 and ADH3 loci that we originally described are now referred to jointly as the ADH class I loci ADH1A, ADH1B and ADH1C. The ADH7 locus is expressed primarily in the stomach and is more related to the class I ADH loci than are the ADH4, ADH5 and ADH6 loci. ADH7 is also involved in conversion of retinol to retinaldehyde (Satre *et al.*, 1994).

Molecular Analyses of Individual Variation of ADH Genes

When DNA probes in the form of cloned segments of the human ADH class I genes became available, we were able to start to use molecular techniques to examine variations in different individuals. The first studies involved finding restriction fragment polymorphisms. Restriction endonucleases are enzymes that cleave DNA at specific sites based on the presence or absence of specific nucleotide sequences at those sites. Cleavage generates fragments of DNA. Mutations with alterations in nucleotide sequence may lead to failure of cleavage at a specific site or to cleavage at new sites. Thus leading to generation of larger or smaller DNA fragments. DNA fragments generated by restriction endonuclease digestion can be separated by electrophoresis on gels e.g. agarose gels. These gels can then be used to generate so-called Southern blots in a process by which DNA is transferred to membranes e.g. nitrocellulose. These membranes can then be hybridized to labeled DNA probes that correspond to a specific gene. In experiments where the DNA probes were labelled with radioactive tags, following hybridization and washing and drying of membranes, the membranes were exposed to photographic film and the pattern of hybridization of probes to the separated restriction endonuclease fragments (DNA fragments) were revealed.

Differences in patterns of hybridization between different individuals when a specific restriction endonuclease was used for digestion, revealed with a specific probe, are referred to as restriction fragment length polymorphisms RFLPs.

Use of Polymerase Chain Reactions (PCR) to Reveal ADH Polymorphisms

Availability of the DNA sequence of a gene and evidence that mutation likely occurs at a particular site in specific individuals permits design of oligonucleotide primers corresponding to DNA sequences that flank the specific site to carry out PCR. In PCR procedures, the DNA to be tested and primers are denatured through exposure to high temperature and this is followed by cooling. Denaturing followed by cooling results in binding of the primers to complementary sequences in the target DNA. Addition of deoxynucleotides triphosphate ATP, TTP, GTP, TTP and DNA polymerase to the reaction allows the synthesis of new DNA strands corresponding to the sequence between the DNA primers.

Sequences differences in ADH class I genes were utilized to develop PCR based assays by Osier et al. (2002) and others.

Availability of PCR greatly facilitated analysis of individual variation in genes. As knowledge of DNA variation was gathered and published, databases were established that documented specific DNA sequence variation at particular locations in the genome. Such sites are documented for example in the dbSNP database at NCBI (www.ncbi.nlm.gov/). The specific nucleotide substitution within the beta ADH (ADH1B) that gives rise to the well documented ADH variant with altered kinetic properties, initially referred to as "atypical ADH", is rs 1229984 in the dbSNP database. The nucleotide substitution at this site leads to an amino acid substitution from arginine to histidine at position 48 in the protein — Arg48His.

Class I ADH Genes and Population Studies

The Arg48His substitution is present in only approximately 10% of individuals of European origin, however it is present in approximately 50% of people of East Asian origins (Osier et al., 2002). The Arg/His substitution was not detected in African or Indian populations. However, another ADH1B polymorphism rs2066702 Arg369Cys is common in individuals from Sub-Saharan Africa (Rao et al., 2007).

In the ADH1C, an interesting polymorphism occurs that is associated with kinetic differences; this is when isoleucine valine substitution Ile349Val occurs. Valine occurs at this site in about 40% of Europeans but it is infrequent in East Asians or in sub-Saharan Africans. ADH1C Ile349 also predominates in individuals from the Indian sub-continent.

It turns out that the Rsa1 restriction fragment length polymorphisms we described in ADH1B are due to an intronic substitution. The frequency of these polymorphisms differs in different populations. This is due to a nucleotide substitution C to T at site 4146 in the gene. The T allele occurs in about 30% of individuals of European origin and about 80% of individuals from East Asia, but it is rare in African populations.

Clinical Relevance of ADH Studies

During the past three decades, many studies have been carried out by different investigators to investigate the role of ADH polymorphisms in propensity to alcoholism. A number of these studies have also included analysis of the variant in mitochondrial aldehyde dehydrogenase ALDH2 discovered by Yoshida et al. in 1983 and known to be present at high frequencies in individuals from South-East Asia. This variant is known to be associated with unpleasant reactions to alcohol consumption. This ALDH2 variant rs671 Glu504Lys occurs in about 20% of individuals of Southeast Asian origin but is rare in Europeans.

The ADH1B variants where arginine at position 48 is replaced by histidine has significantly altered kinetics and is associated with increased and rapid generation of aldehyde and its side effects including significant facial flushing, sweating and may lead to a fall in blood pressure.

Way et al. (2015) reported that the presence of the variant allele in rs1229984 with histidine at position 48 does occur in a low percentage of individuals in British and Irish populations and has a protective effect against alcoholism.

Holmes et al. (2014) reported results of a comprehensive study of 261,991 individuals of European descent and noted that individuals with the variant allele in rs122984 (A on forward sequence, T on reverse) had a lower frequency of binge drinking and a higher abstention rate. These individuals also had a more favorable cardiovascular profile including lower systolic blood pressure and lower body mass index. In addition, these individuals also manifested decreased risk of coronary heart disease.

ADH variants have also been studied relative to the risk for development of specific forms of cancer. In addition, investigations were undertaken to analyze harmful effects to the fetus of alcohol consumption during pregnancy and the possible roles of alcohol variants in altering risk.

High alcohol consumption has been associated with increased risk for a number of different cancers, including head and neck cancers such as oral cavity, pharynx and larynx (Zhang et al., 2015) reported individuals with the His allele at position 48 in ADH1B are at decreased risk for head and neck cancer, likely because they are less likely to be exposed to alcohol.

Fetal Alcohol Exposure

The hazards to the fetus of heavy alcohol consumption by pregnant women were documented in 1976 by Smith et al. The effects on the fetus of moderate alcohol consumption by pregnant women were reported by Lewis et al. in 2012. Their studies were based on analyses in the Avon Birth Cohort. They studied the children of mothers who had moderate alcohol consumption during pregnancy and children of mothers who abstained from alcohol consumption during pregnancy. They determined that specific genetic variants in ADH class 1 genes in children influenced the risk of intellectual impairment in offspring of mothers who had moderate alcohol consumption during pregnancy. These genetic variants in children had no effect on IQ in children of mothers who consumed no alcohol during pregnancy.

Of particular interest is the fact that two of the variants that occurred in children and were significantly associated with intellectual impairment in alcohol-exposed children occurred in the ADH1A gene. The ADH1A gene encodes the predominant form of alcohol dehydrogenase expressed in fetal liver from early fetal life onwards (Smith et al., 1971). One significantly associated allele in children occurred in ADH1B and another occurred in the ADH7 gene. ADH 7 is not a class I ADH. It is associated with metabolism of several alcohols and also with conversion of the alcohol retinol to retinaldehyde. The latter plays a significant role during development.

Significance values ($p=$) for the association of variants in children and risk of intellectual impairment following fetal alcohol exposure are listed below:

ADH1A   rs2866151 $p = 0.004$

ADH1A   rs975833 $p = 0.03$

ADH1B   rs4147536 $p = 0.05$

ADH7   rs284799 $p = 0.003$

A different allele is associated with maternal tolerance of binge drinking, namely the wild type allele of ADH rs1229984 (A on forward reaction, T on reverse) Arg46. Binge drinking in mothers can be associated with significant damage to the fetus.

26 Gene Mapping and Somatic Cell Genetics

Following the period in 1965–1966 when I undertook studies concentrating on nuclei, chromatin and chromosomes in human cells and took courses in biochemistry and plant genetics, I mentioned my interest in carrying out work in human genetics to a faculty member known for his work on bacteriophages. He dismissed my interest with the comment: "You cannot do genetics in humans, their generation time is too long". This put-down comment was in fact inaccurate.

Human Gene Mapping

The first form of gene mapping carried out in humans involved analyzing the occurrence of a specific phenotypic characteristic in different members of successive generations in a family. Through such family studies, color blindness was shown to be passed on through unaffected females to half of their sons. Wilson (1911) reported that the gene determining color blindness mapped to the human X chromosome.

In human genetics, there had for many years been a goal to link particular genetic diseases to particular markers that occurred in disease affected members in a family and were absent in unaffected family members. Linkage depended on analysis of the inheritance of a specific phenotype and inheritance of specific markers that demonstrated detectable variations. Initially, most markers used were protein markers. However, there were few protein markers available and few examples emerged of diseases that could be linked to genetic markers. The first linkage of a human disease to a genetic marker was the discovery by Renwick and Lawler (1955) that the ABO blood group locus was linked to a genetic disorder nail-patella syndrome. The first example of mapping of a human polymorphic protein to a human chromosome occurred in 1968 when Donahue *et al.* reported that in a specific family, a specific allele of the Duffy blood group segregated with an unusual cytogenetic variant on chromosome 1.

Somatic Cell Hybrids

In 1967, Weiss and Green first reported that human and mouse cells could undergo fusion in the presence of Sendai virus. Separation of hybrid cells from mouse cells was achieved by the use of rodent cells that could be selected against by certain chemicals or by specific culture conditions, so that unfused rodent cells died. For example, rodent cells for fusion were generated that lacked a specific enzyme and could be selected against. Human lymphocytes were often used in fusion experiments. Following fusion, hybrid clones were grown as cells attached to the surface of culture vessels. The unfused, unattached human lymphocytes were quickly removed as culture medium was removed and replaced with fresh medium. The hybrid cells that resulted from fusion could be cultured and they were shown to lose human chromosomes in successive waves.

In these hybrid cells, mouse and human chromosomes could be distinguished and identification of specific human chromosomes was facilitated by the introduction of chromosome banding methods, including those developed by Caspersson *et al.* (1970) and by Seabright in1972. A major advance in distinguishing human and mouse chromosomes came through the introduction of the Giemsa 11 staining technique by Friend *et al.* in 1976. When Giemsa stain at pH 11 was used to stain chromosomes spread on glass slides, the mouse and human chromosomes differed in their staining intensity.

Gel electrophoresis of extracts of hybrid cells followed by application of specific staining methods enabled the detection of rodent and human forms of specific enzymes. The human and rodent forms of a specific enzyme could often be readily distinguished because they had charge differences and migrated differently on electrophoresis. The retention of specific human enzymes or proteins could then be correlated with the retention of specific human chromosomes in specific hybrid clones.

Mapping of specific genes to human chromosomes progressed very well following the introduction of somatic cell hybrid methods.

Human gene mapping conferences were held regularly following the first mapping conference in 1973.

An important breakthrough that facilitated generation of somatic cell hybrids was the report in 1975 by Pontecorvo that the chemical poly-ethylene glycol could be used to facilitate cell fusion. Thus it became no longer necessary to culture Sendai virus in chicken eggs in order to obtain reagent to generate hybrids.

My own adventures in somatic cell genetics began in 1974 when I was a post-doctoral fellow in the laboratory of Dr. Phil Gold at the Montreal General Hospital at McGill University in Canada. Dr. Gold encouraged me to develop and use somatic cell hybrids to map genes that encode proteins involved in human immune function. Through work on cell fusion, hybrid selection, characterization of the human content of cloned hybrid cells, and through use of antibodies, we were able to map the human beta2mi-croglobulin protein to human chromosome 15. This was surprising, since beta2microglobulin was complexed with the HLA antigens that mapped to human chromosome 6.

I continued studies aimed at mapping genes to human chromosomes as a junior faculty member at Mount Sinai Hospital in New York and was fortunate enough to be able to start attending the Human Gene Mapping Workshops held in various cities in North America and Europe.

When I joined the faculty at the University of California, Irvine in 1981, I continued gene mapping research and was fortunate enough to be able to collaborate with John Wasmuth on mapping projects. John had particular expertise in the development and use of temperature sensitive Chinese Hamster ovary (CHO) cell lines to produce somatic cell hybrids (Cirullo et al., 1983). One of the advantages of use of these CHO cell lines was that the hybrid cells generated from them retained very few human chromosomes.

As molecular biology and molecular genetics expertise progressed it became possible to map DNA probes and DNA corresponding to specific genes to human chromosomes.

27 Catching up on Developments in Molecular Genetics through the 1960s and 1970s

When I joined the faculty at the University of California, Irvine in 1981 and had the opportunity to collaborate with faculty and students in a molecular genetics unit within the Department of Microbiology in the Medical School, I realized that it was time to catch up on development in molecular genetics. I spent time reviewing the history and reading the literature.

In 1953, Watson and Crick reported the structure of DNA. This structure was derived primarily through detailed X-Ray crystallographic studies and through prior knowledge that DNA was composed of purine and pyrimidine nucleotides attached to deoxyribose phosphate residues. They reported that the key aspects of the structure included the existence of two helical chains coiled around the same axis. The chains were held together by purine and pyrimidine bases and specifically through weak hydrogen bonds between the bases. Furthermore, they demonstrated that bonding occurred specifically between adenine (purine) and thymine (pyrimidine) and between guanine (purine) and cytosine (pyrimidine). The bases were therefore positioned on the inside of the helix and the phosphate residues on deoxyribose were positioned on the outside.

An oft quoted sentence from the Watson and Crick 1963 paper includes the important observation:

"It has not escaped our notice that the specific pairing we have postulated immediately suggests a possible copying mechanism for the genetic material".

Intense Efforts on Molecular Biology followed Discovery of the DNA Structure

In 1960, Doty et al. reported information on methods to separate complementary strands of DNA and factors that facilitated recombining of DNA strands. They outlined methods to promote denaturing and renaturing of DNA and the degree and extent of homology required for two DNA strands to recombine. These methods were to become key factors in genetic analyses.

In 1961, Brenner, Jacob and Meselson were the first to report that while genetic information for proteins is encoded in DNA, the actual assembly of proteins occurs on ribosomes and that an intermediate exists between DNA and proteins. They designated this intermediate messenger RNA (mRNA) and they established that this unstable intermediate molecule carried information from DNA in genes to the 70S ribosome. Ribosomes were shown to be non-specialized structures that synthesized proteins dictated by the messenger RNA that represented a copy of the gene.

Detailed studies by Nirenberg, Leder and others (1964) established how the mRNA code specified the amino acids that were progressively added to the peptide chain during protein synthesis. These investigators reported that specific triplet trinucleotide codons in the presence of transfer RNA molecules (that each carried a specific amino acid) generated polypeptides with defined sequence that reflected the sequence in the gene.

By 1966, the genetic code that specifies synthesis of proteins that contain the 20 natural amino acids had been determined. The triplet code was shown to be degenerate, in that the last nucleotide in particular varied in some cases, so that some amino acids had more than one codon; one example was phenylalanine that could be specified by the RNA code UUU or by UUC.

In 1966 Crick wrote:

"Thus protein is written in a twenty letter language, nucleic acid is written in a four letter language. The genetic code is the dictionary that connects the two languages".

Enzymes and the Molecular Revolution

Polymerases

Polymerases were used from the early stages of molecular biology research on to the present. In 1956, Arthur Kornberg discovered DNA polymerase 1, the enzyme that can synthesize a new strand of DNA in the presence of a DNA template and a mixture of trinucleotides (that contain deoxyribose as the sugar residues), adenosine triphosphate (ATP), cytosine triphosphate (CTP), guanine triphosphate (GTP) and thymine triphosphate (TTP).

    Different forms of polymerase proved useful; later in DNA sequencing a specific fragment of a polymerase from *E. coli*, Klenow fragment, proved particularly useful.

    RNA polymerase was co-discovered in 1959 by two groups that include Weiss in one group and Hurwitz in another group. RNA polymerase, also known as DNA dependent RNA polymerase can synthesize an RNA strand using a DNA template and ribonucleotides (that contain ribose as the sugar residues), adenosine-5'triphosphate phosphate (ATP), guanosine triphosphate (GTP), cytosine-5-triphosphate (CTP) and uridine-5-monophosphate (UTP).

Reverse Transcriptase

In 1970, Temin & Mizutani and Baltimore reported discovery of an enzyme that could generate DNA corresponding to an RNA sequence. This enzyme RNA transcriptase enabled generation of CDNA (copy DNA) from messenger RNA. These DNA fragments could then be cloned into vectors including plasmids and bacteriophages.

Restriction Endonucleases

In 1970, Smith and Wilcox made key contributions to characterization of restriction endonucleases and to the definition of their cleavage sites. Restriction endonucleases cleave double stranded DNA at specific 4–8 base-pair locations. Restriction endonucleases can be used to generate fragments of DNA.

Following digestion of DNA with restriction endonucleases, electro-phoresis and application of DNA binding dyes (such as ethidium bromide) specific patterns of DNA can be discerned.

Ligases

Ligase enzymes proved to be essential in cloning for insertion of DNA fragments into DNA of vectors.

Southern Blots

Southern (1975) described a method whereby DNA fragments separated by electrophoresis on agarose could be transferred to nitrocellulose matrix filter paper. Specially treated filters could then be exposed to radioactively labeled DNA probes (e.g. gene fragments). Subsequently, bound probes could be detected through exposure of the treated and DNA hybridized nitrocellulose filters to photographic film.

DNA Sequencing

Sanger (1977) published a method to determine the nucleotide sequences; his method was based on the sequential synthesis of new strands of DNA in the presence of DNA polymerase trinucleotides and a DNA template. In 1977, Maxam and Gilbert published a different sequencing method based on chemical degradation of DNA. Shortly thereafter, Sanger introduced a modification to his sequencing method. This modification involved the addition of dideoxynucleotide triphosphates (ddNTPs), that lack hydroxyl groups at their 3' residues of deoxyribose units, so that addition of a subsequent nucleotide cannot be added to the DNA chain being synthesized.

For sequencing of human DNA, segments of DNA were most frequently cloned into a bacteriophage vector. A specific oligonucleo-tide sequence, usually selected to match the bacteriophage sequence near the site into which foreign DNA was cloned, was used to initiate DNA synthesis in the presence of polymerase, deoxynucleotides (CTP, GTP, TTP, ATP including radiolabeled ATP), p32ATP dideoxynucleotides. For each experiment, four different tubes were set up; each tube contained a different dideoxynucleotide (ddATP, ddTTP, ddCTP, or ddGTP). The chain of sequence terminated when the ddNTP was added to the reaction and termination of sequence of a specific fragment occurred at that point.

Following the sequencing reactions, products were electrophoresed on denaturing polyacrylamide gels to separate sequence fragments of different lengths. The gels were subsequently dried and exposed to photographic film. The successive termination of sequence in fragments could then be discerned. The sequence could then be read as a ladder.

The Impact of the Molecular Cloning Manual of Sambrook, Fritsch and Maniatis

In considering the methodologies developed to facilitate molecular genetic studies it is important that homage be paid to Sambrook, Fritch and Maniatis, who published extensive manuals of laboratory methods. These manuals entitled "Molecular Cloning" were first used for courses in eukaryotic cloning given at Cold Spring Harbor Laboratories. The researchers and administration at Cold Spring Harbor deserves particular acknowledgement for facilitating the spreading of knowledge and expertise in biology and its application to problems in biology and medicine.

It is also important to emphasize that reagents, including enzymes and biochemical reagents, became more readily available to researchers through growth of enterprising companies that grew up stimulated by the progress in recombinant DNA methods.

Interrupted Genes

Independent reports by Sharp and by Roberts (www.nobelprize.org/nobel_prizes/medicine/laureates/1993/press.html) in 1977 revealed the first evidence that genes of higher organisms differed from genes in bacteriophages in that they contained coding regions and non-coding regions. Gilbert (1978) summarized the finding and reported: "The Gene is a mosaic of expressed sequences held in a matrix of silent DNA, an intronic matrix". Gilbert also emphasized that the dogma of one gene one polypeptide chain had disappeared. Transcription from a particular gene could lead to the generation of many polypeptide chains and that the different chains could have related or different functions. Gilbert also perceived that different splicing patterns of exons could play roles in the different gene expression patterns that occurred during differentiation of multi-cellular organisms. He also perceived the important implications of introns and exons for evolution, noting that portions of introns could give rise to new exons: "extra-material is scattered through the genome to be called into action at any time".

In 2013, on the sixtieth anniversary of the publication of the paper describing the Watson and Crick DNA structure model, Doolittle and twelve genomic biologists selected key advances that followed that publication. The one advance that they mutually selected as paradigm shifting was publication of evidence that eukaryotic genes were interrupted. Gravel emphasized that the occurrence of introns and delineation of splicing mechanisms that removed introns and discovery of alternative splicing of specific genes has far reaching implications. He emphasized that Gilbert had rapidly recognized that alternative splicing would increase protein diversity and alternative splicing could drive differentiation. A number of other investigators including Keren et al. (2010) had demonstrated the important implications of introns for evolution.

Increased availability of DNA and RNA sequencing analyses have revealed that defects in splicing are key factors in the causation of a number of human genetic diseases.

In recent years, important insights have been gained into the structure and function of spliceosomes, the complexes that carry out splicing. In addition, the composition and activities of splicing regulatory factors, including specific nucleotide sequences and specific RNA binding factors, have been gained (Fu and Ares, 2014).

Incorporation of DNA Technology into Human Gene Mapping and Linkage Studies

DNA markers for human gene mapping and linkage studies

As molecular techniques (including DNA cloning) developed, DNA polymorphisms were described and were intensely investigated -as markers for linkage studies and chromosome mapping. DNA polymorphisms included variation between individuals in restriction endonuclease cleavage sites. These variations were referred to as restriction fragment length polymorphisms (RFLPs). Differences in restriction endonuclease cleavage sites led to the generation of DNA fragments of different sizes that could be demonstrated, following electrophoresis of restriction endonuclease digested DNA on gels, southern blotting of the gels and hybridization of the blots with specific DNA probes. DNA probes used for hybridization were segments of DNA from different regions of the genome. In some experiments, the DNA probes used for hybridization were derived through cloning of DNA derived from specific human chromosomes. Specific human chromosomes could be separated by a number of different techniques, including fluorescence activated cell sorting.

In 1983, Gusella and colleagues reported their discovery that a specific DNA probe derived from human chromosome 4 detected a specific restriction fragment length polymorphic variant that was linked to the Huntington disease phenotype in two separate pedigrees. Huntington disease is a dominantly inherited disease that leads to severe movement abnormalities, psychiatric symptoms and intellectual deterioration. Manifestations commence usually between the third and fifth decades of life. The report by Gusella *et al.* represented the first evidence that DNA markers could be used to map human disease.

DNA Amplification through use of the Polymerase Chain Reaction (PCR)

In 1986, Mullis *et al.* reported that the reciprocal interaction of two oligonucleotide probes in the presence of nucleotides and heat resistant DNA polymerase could amplify the DNA sequence between the two oligonucleotide primers. The oligonucleotide primers should be designed so that one primer corresponded to a sequence at the 5'end of one strand of the double stranded DNA segment to be amplified and the 2nd oligonucleotide primer hybridized to the 5'-end of the corresponding reciprocal strand in the DNA segment.

Successive cycles of heating and cooling were required to promote the reaction. During heating, the double stranded DNA opened and allowed hybridization of the oligonucleotide primer. Subsequent cooling was required for the synthesis of new DNA. Under appropriate conditions, the polymerase chain reaction led to synthesis of large amounts of DNA corresponding to the sequence between the primers. The amplified DNA could be used in studies to detect nucleotide sequence and nucleotide variants in the specific DNA segment. The amplified DNA could also be cloned into vectors.

Discovery of Polymorphic Markers through Application of PCR Technology

Other markers that detected individual variation were developed. These DNA markers included segments of human DNA that demonstrated variation in the number of nucleotide repeats they contained.

Microsatellite repeat markers included segments of DNA with blocks of dinucleotide repeats, often CA or GT repeats. The exact number of repeats in a specific DNA segment differed in different individuals, however the number of repeats in a specific DNA segment followed Mendelian inheritance patterns. The highly polymorphic microsatellite repeat markers were very useful for linkage analysis.

It was also critically important to map the individual microsatellite repeat markers to specific human chromosomes and this was possible through PCR, using somatic cell hybrids that contained specific human chromosomes. In some experiments, sorted human chromosomes were used in microsatellite repeat based PCR experiments.

Investigators collaborated to construct a framework map of highly polymorphic markers across the genome to facilitate linkage analysis in families. In 1996, Dib et al. reported availability of the Genethon Human Linkage Map of 5,264 highly polymorphic microsatellite markers that mapped across the genome.

Physical Mapping of Markers to Chromosomes

In situ hybridization

In situ hybridization methods involved the hybridization of labelled DNA probes to microscope slides with spreads of human chromosomes, usually chromosomes in the metaphase stage of cell division. In situ hybridization of probes to chromosomes was greatly enhanced by the introduction of a modification reported by Harper and Chan in 1986. They reported that addition of dextran sulfate to the hybridization solution enhanced reaction of probe with chromosomal DNA. In addition, *in situ* hybridization was expedited when fluorescently labeled nucleotides became available and these could be used along with DNA polymerase to generate labeled DNA probes.

Advances in Nucleic Acid Sequencing Techniques

In 1987, Hood *et al.* described methods for automated sequencing. Key to automation was the introduction of fluorescent labeled nucleotides that enabled detection of labeled DNA by lasers. Initial automated sequencing efforts were based primarily on Sanger sequencing methods. The first automated sequencer was developed by Lloyd Smith and introduced into the market by ABI.

28 The Human Genome Project and Advances in Genetics and Genomics

In 1988, the National Research Council (NRC) in the USA recommended "mounting a special effort to map and sequence the human genome". They recommended development of maps of polymorphic markers and maps of coding DNA segments in initial efforts (McKusick, 2006). They also recommended emphasis on technological developments related to mapping and sequencing. The NRC proposed support of medium-sized multi-disciplinary centers. In such centers, they suggested that interactions between biologists, physicists, engineers and information scientists should take place.

In 1988 the director of the National Institutes of Health USA James Wyngaarden created the Human Genome Research Center. The US Department of Energy also established a Genomics Center.

The Human Genome Project (HGP) was launched in the USA in 1990 and it became an international effort, with mapping and sequencing efforts carried out in several European countries and in Japan and China.

In addition to the government supported efforts, a privately funded Human Genome project was initiated in the USA under the direction of Craig Venter and the company Celera.

The underlying design of efforts differed somewhat between the government sponsored (NIH) and the privately sponsored project in the USA. The NIH projects selected mapping as a first approach, with development of a framework map of sequenced segments throughout the genome that was then followed by expanding outward from the sequenced site. The Celera efforts concentrated initially on sequenced cloned cDNA representing expressed sequence labeled as Expressed Sequence Tags (ESTs).

Essential to the Human Genome Sequencing project was the development of libraries of human DNA cloned into vectors that could accommodate large segments of DNA including genomic DNA. The Bac vector proved particularly useful for this cloning (Leonardo and Sedivy, 1990). Specific Bac clones were characterized by the fingerprint pattern of their restriction endonuclease digested DNA and by identification of their chromosome map position. Specific clones were positioned by fluorescence in situ hybridization to human chromosomes.

Early Fruits of the HGP: A Map of Sequence Tagged Sites

An early product of the NIH funded efforts was production of a physical map of the genome based on sequenced tagged sites. These sequence tagged sites did not necessarily map within genes. They represented segments of DNA mapped to specific locations through the genome and the segments could be analyzed by PCR. The physical map described by Hudson et al. in 1995 comprised 15,086 loci in the genome. These sequenced tags were identified through sequencing libraries of genomic DNA cloned in vectors.

In addition to the presence of unique sequence segments in the human genome, sequencing of Bac clones containing sequences from across the genome revealed the occurrence of repeated sequence elements. Some regions of the genome were particularly rich in repetitive sequences. In addition, there was evidence that elements with specific sequences were duplicated in different regions of the genome.

Draft Sequence of the Human Genome

In 2001, a draft sequence of the human genome was produced. Ultimately, production of the draft sequence assembly combined sequence data from the public effort and the private efforts. The draft sequence still contained gaps and further efforts were required to improve accuracy.

Sequencing of genomic regions of different individuals led to the identification of 104 million mapped single nucleotide variants (polymorphisms) — SNPs that could be used for linkage studies to follow inheritance of diseases and for identifications of specific individuals and their family relationships.

Venter *et al.* (2001) reported that fewer than 1% of the single nucleotide polymorphisms (SNPs) impacted protein function. They noted, however, that thousands of variants were estimated to contribute to protein variation.

The number of protein coding loci in the human genome was reported in 2001 to be approximately 30,000. That number turned out to be lower than anticipated and to be only twice as large as the expressed gene number in lower organisms, including *Drosophila*. However, the protein loci in human were found to be more complex than those present in lower organisms. The complex protein encoding loci in human could each give rise to numerous gene products.

Next-Generation Sequencing Methods

Massively parallel sequencing

Following on from the development of sequencing with fluorescent nucleotides, massively parallel sequencing methods were developed. These sequencing methods involve shearing of genomic DNA into fragments approximately 300 base pairs in size, and ligation of adapters at each end of the fragments. The libraries of fragments are then amplified in polymerase chains reactions (PCR). Different systems vary in the following steps. The amplified fragments may be bound to beads by virtue of affinity of the adapters to coating on the beads. In some systems, beads are then immobilized in individual wells of a fiber optic slide. Each well contains reagents for carrying out the sequencing reaction with DNA polymerase and nucleotides (ddNTPs); each of the 4 nucleotides have a different colored fluorescent tag. Sequential addition of nucleotides to the growing DNA strand is monitored by laser light. Each individual DNA strand captured in a well is sequenced from both ends and each strand is sequenced multiple times. The short sequence reads generated are then aligned to the reference DNA sequence through specific bioinformatics programs.

The advantages of massively parallel sequencing include accuracy of sequencing. A disadvantage of massively parallel sequencing is that the sequence reads are short.

Third Generation Sequencing Methods

Third generation sequencing methods include single molecule sequencing of larger DNA fragments. In the PacBio sequencing system a circularized DNA strand diffuses into a unit on a chip. DNA polymerase and fluorescent nucleotides are immobilized in each unit. Each nucleotide is sequentially added to synthesize a new DNA strand. The addition of each specific nucleotide changes the light wavelength to a different degree. The sequential changes in light wavelength are sequentially measured and plotted. PacBio sequencing can generate kilobase sequence lengths.

The ability to read long lengths of sequences facilitates closing gaps in the sequence. It also facilitates reading through stretches of nucleotide repeats in the DNA sequencing. In addition, reading of long lengths of sequences facilitates defining the exact sequences of genes that share blocks of homology but that also have non-homologous regions (Rhoads and Au, 2015).

Nanopore Sequencing

Nanopore sequencing is a new development in single molecule sequencing. In this method, single molecules of DNA are forced through a pore in a solid state material. The pore is usually one nanometer in size. The solid state material is immersed in an electric current conducting medium. As each nucleotide passes through the nanopore it alters the electric current and each of the four nucleotides alter electric current to a different degree. The alteration in electric current is measured and plotted. Commercialization of nanopore sequencing has been achieved by a number of companies including Oxford Nanopore Technologies.

Analysis of Functional Elements in the Genome

Following on the initial Human Genome Project and generation of a Draft sequence, the ENCODE project commenced. This project was designed to examine the function of the approximately 3 billion bases in the Human Genome. Earlier studies on the function of the genome concentrated on specific individual genes. The ENCODE project sought to provide more comprehensive information on functional elements in the genome. The

ENCODE project revealed that the human genome is extensively transcribed and that transcripts were derived not only from protein coding regions but also from non-protein coding regions. In some cases, transcripts initiated in non-protein coding regions overlapped with transcripts from protein coding regions. In addition, the extensive complexity of transcription regulation was revealed. This complexity involved not only regulatory sequences within the genome, it also involved the state of chromatin, the histone matrix around which DNA is wound.

The ENCODE project also provided further information on DNA sequence sites in the genome where transcription is initiated, on the transcription factors that bind to these sites and the state of chromatin at these sites (ENCODE project consortium 2012).

Chromatin Architecture and Transcription

Chromatin is composed of histone-rich nucleosomes around which DNA strands are coiled, and of linker fibers between nucleosomes. The degree of packing of nucleosomes in chromatin, whether they are closely packed or whether chromatin has an open structure, greatly impacts transcription. Initiation of transcription of DNA occurs more commonly in open chromatin, where spaces occur between nucleosomes. Open chromatin can be identified through its greater sensitivity to digestion with the enzyme DNAse 1. This fact has facilitated identification of transcription initiation sites in the genome. Other important factors that regulate DNA transcription are the type and extent of modification of specific amino acids in histone chromatin. These modifications primarily involve addition or subtraction of methyl groups and acetyl groups to specific amino acids, particularly to lysine in chromatin. Key elements in transcription are specific sequence elements in DNA to which transcription factors bind. In the ENCODE project, catalogs of transcription factors and their DNA binding sites were developed.

Non-protein-coding RNA

Non-protein-coding RNA includes the earlier characterized RNA forms such as ribosomal RNA and transfer RNA, and microRNAs and small nucleolar RNAs. The ENCODE project revealed the existence of non-protein-coding

RNA transcripts including long non-protein-coding transcripts, lncRNAs. The pervasive transcription of the genome established that the genome was not comprised of long tracts of "Junk DNA" as had been previously suggested.

Relevance of Information on the Human Genome Sequence and of Transcription Information for Clinical Medicine

Genetic information can be valuable for disease diagnosis, for health management and for family planning. It is clear, however, that interpretation of the importance of specific sequence changes remains challenging in many situations. The sheer numbers of variants in sequence in each person's genome are staggering. In addition, the frequencies of specific variants vary in different populations. Ongoing efforts in correlation of genomic sequence information with phenotypic findings and disease manifestations and the development of accessible information in databases remain critical elements for progress. In addition, ongoing efforts to correlate specific sequence changes with alterations in protein stability and function remain critical.

Microarrays

Availability of gene and genome sequence information and technology development enabled the development of microarrays. On these arrays, oligonucleotides representing individual gene and genome segments were imprinted onto a solid matrix in a grid pattern. Fluorescently labeled samples derived from patient DNA or messenger RNA from blood or tissues could be hybridized to the microarrays. Following washing to remove unbound DNA or RNA, a signal emitted by the bound DNA or RNA could then be detected by laser scanning of the arrays.

Microarrays are used to analyze human genomic DNA for the presence of deletions or deletions of genomic segments. Microarrays and blood or tissue derived mRNA are also used to analyze gene expression in tissues and in tumors.

Microarrays of oligonucleotide sequences corresponding to specific nucleotide polymorphisms (including single nucleotide polymorphisms and microsatellite repeat polymorphisms) known to map to specific genomic regions are used to analyze DNA variation. In some cases, such microarray analysis is carried out in families, to identify markers and genomic segments that co-segregate with specific phenotypes including diseases.

Analysis of a Specific Gene or Analysis of a Gene Panel

Diagnostic testing may involve microarray analyses, or sequencing that covers all exons or the entire genome. In some cases, a more targeted study is carried out that involves microarray analyses or sequencing of a single gene or of a panel of genes known to frequently be mutated in disorders with specific phenotypic manifestations.

Whole Exome or Whole Genome Sequencing

A number of clinically significant diagnoses have been made and reported in cases of rare gene based disorders. In a number of these cases, multiple studies carried out prior to sequencing had failed to reveal diagnoses.

It is clear, however, that interpretation of the clinical significance of specific sequence changes remains challenging in many situations. As a first assessment it is important in the cases of putative single gene disorders to determine the frequency of the sequence variant found in healthy individuals in a healthy population. A number of databases are useful in this regard, e.g. ExAC and 1000 genomes. In considering which variants are likely to be significant in contributing to disease pathogenesis. Variants that are not common in the general population may also have been encountered in other individuals and be documented in NCBI databases, including dbSNP and ClinVar. The specific nature of the variant is important to consider. Sequence variants that are documented as leading to loss of function of the protein are particularly important. Splice site variants are also important to consider. Missense variants that change the amino acid at a particular site in the protein may or may not be significant in altering protein function. In some cases, it is possible to gather information concerning the impact of specific mutations on a protein through consultation with databases (SIFT, PolyPhen).

It is also important that sequence changes that are apparently clinically significant be confirmed by direct sequencing, e.g. Sanger sequencing. Sequence information from parents and from affected and unaffected siblings is often necessary to assess the significance of sequence changes.

In addition, biochemical assays to analyze the functional impact of specific gene mutations on protein function and structure are important. Much work remains to be done in documenting specific gene defects, and in correlating specific gene defects and the phenotypic alterations observed and associated biochemical and physiological changes.

Mutation Types and Consequences

The most damaging DNA mutations that most frequently led to disease are defined as loss of function mutations. Loss of function mutations can include mutations at the transcription stop site, that leads to abnormally short or abnormally long transcripts. Splice site variants may also lead to loss of function; splice site mutations lead to transcripts that are missing exons or to transcripts that fail to excise introns. Deletions of nucleotides within exons or addition of nucleotides that alter the reading frame of transcripts and alter codons for amino acids are also damaging.

In Mendelian dominant diseases, damaging mutations as described above can lead to disease if they occur in a specific gene located on a single member of a homologous chromosome pair. For example, specific mutation in the TSC2 gene on one member of the chromosome 16 pair can lead to the disease tuberous sclerosis.

Recessive diseases result if damaging mutations occur in a specific gene on each member of a specific pair of homologous chromosomes. For example, damaging mutations in PAH genes on both members of the chromosome 12 pair lead to phenylketonuria. In recessive disease, the disease causing mutation may be the same on each of the two chromosomes (homozygous mutations), or different damaging mutations in the same gene on each member of the chromosome pair may occur and lead to disease. For example, a stop site mutation may occur in the PAH gene on one chromosome 12 and a splice site mutation may occur in the PAH gene on the other chromosome 12, the patient is then a compound heterozygote for damaging mutations.

Loss of function mutations in both members of a gene pair are sometimes referred to as gene knockouts.

An unexpected finding of comprehensive DNA sequencing was that loss of function mutations or gene knockouts sometimes occurred in healthy individuals. In sequencing in the Icelandic population including 2,636 healthy individuals, Sulem *et al.* (2015) reported that 7.7% of individuals sequenced had complete knockout of a single gene due to loss of function mutations. The main category of genes that demonstrated knockouts were olfactory receptor genes. Of the 1,171 genes that showed knockout, 26 of the genes had previously been reported as being involved in diseases.

It is important to emphasize, however, that to completely assess the significance of the knockout findings it will be important to determine if the specific gene was knocked out in all tissue or if knockout occurred only in DNA derived from the most frequently sequenced tissue, namely blood cells. Sulem *et al.* (2015) emphasized the importance of follow-up studies.

Genome-wide Association Studies

The wide distribution of single nucleotide variants throughout the genome was used in studies to identify genomic regions important in the etiology of common complex diseases in adults including diabetes, cardiovascular diseases and late onset neurodegenerative diseases. Such studies became known as genome-wide association studies, GWAS. In 2013, Manolio reported that GWAS had identified approximately 2,000 definitive associations with 300 complex diseases. However, Manolio pointed out that each associated variant contributed to risk in a very small degree. The presence of an associated variant was of very little value in predicting disease risk in a particular individual.

Interesting information however emerged from GWAS; these studies provided insight into specific pathogenic pathways involved in specific complex common diseases. Another important finding is that associated variants for complex common diseases are most commonly located in regulatory regions of the genome and not in the protein coding regions of the genome. Regulatory regions included enhancer segments of the genome, promoter regions and transcription factor binding sites.

Impact of Gene Interactions

Studies of the effect of a specific variant on phenotype and studies of the association of variants with disease occurrence most often fail to take into account the fact the products of genes interact and that different genes may be co-regulated. Studies on the effects of a genetic variant also fail to take into account the fact that a specific biochemical process in the body may be carried out by a series of homologous genes.

Failure to consider gene interactions may be particularly relevant in complex common diseases. Investigators often point out that taking family history into account often leads to assessment that a particular common complex disease has high heritability but that only a small proportion of the heritability can be explained by variants identified in GWAS. Zuk et al. (2012) proposed that missing heritability could be explained by interactions between genes and perhaps by the existence of variants not yet identified.

Genome-wide Association Studies and Information on Susceptibility to Medication Toxicity

A number of genome-wide association studies have provided insight into variants that are associated with abnormal responses to particular medications. One example includes variants that influence occurrence of side effects to treatment with the drug Ribavirin used in the treatment of hepatitis C infections. GWAS revealed that variants in the gene that encodes inosine triphosphatase, an enzyme involved in purine metabolism, reduce activity of the enzyme and increase side-effects of the drug Thompson et al. (2010). GWAS on patients who develop muscle weakness in response to statins, used to treat increased lipid levels, revealed that variants in the gene SLCO1B1 occurred. The SLCO1B1 encoded protein is a solute carrier transporter (Search Collaborative Group, 2008).

DNA Analysis in Forensics

In the area of forensics, DNA analysis can provide accurate identification of victims and suspects. However, the methods of collection of samples for testing and avoidance of contamination of samples from one individual with samples from another individual is critical.

The most reliable forms of DNA analysis for forensic purposes include analysis of short tandem nucleotide repeat polymorphisms at different locations in the genome. The number of genome locations analyzed varies between 13 and 33.

Polymerase chain reaction methodologies enable analysis of trace quantities of DNA. However, this increased sensitivity can lead to problems since trace quantities of DNA can be left on items for long periods and may have been deposited on items long before a crime took place.

DNA Analysis in Cancer

The key goal in analysis of DNA mutations that arise in tumors is to identify those mutations that are significant in promoting growth, invasiveness and metastasis of tumors. Vogelstein (2013) emphasized that although specific mutations act as driver mutations, all mutations in tumors are not driver mutations. It is also useful to identify specific genes that tend to act as driver mutations in different types of tumors. Driver mutations in the TP53 transcription factor occur in a number of different types of cancer. Mutations in genes defined as oncogenes (e.g. RAS, KRAS and BRAF) also occur in a number of different cancers. Driver gene mutations often impact genes that play roles in cell signaling pathways, in genes that influence cell cycle and in genes that impact regulation of gene expression.

In addition to identifying driver gene mutations that are known to occur frequently in tumors (recurrent mutations), it is also important to have methods that detect non-recurrent mutations and mutations specific to a particular tumor.

The goal is to identify mutations that may be targeted by specific therapies.

DNA sequencing of tumors can also be useful in revealing certain chromosome rearrangements and unusual gene fusions in tumors. A number of tumor specific gene fusions play important roles in promoting tumor growth and invasiveness.

DNA sequencing has, however, revealed that DNA in malignant tumors continues to undergo mutations leading to heterogeneity both at the primary site and in metastases. This continual mutation and heterogeneity frequently leads tumors to become resistant to targeted therapies that initially seemed effective.

Hereditary Cancer Syndromes

Germline mutations, including inherited mutations, have been identified as predisposing to certain cancer types. Examples include germline mutations in DNA repair genes that predispose to colon cancer. The predisposing mutations are usually present in heterozygous form in the blood cells of carriers, and second hit mutations occur in the tumor. Identification of mutations that increase the risk of certain cancers in carrier individuals indicate that these individuals should be frequently screened to detect cancer at an early stage.

Analysis of Gene Expression in Tumors

A number of different factors impact gene expression in tumors. These include DNA mutations, structural genomic changes including deletion or duplications of gene-containing segments, and genomic rearrangements in tumors that lead to the generations of fusion genes. In addition, epigenetic changes including the degree of methylation of cytosine residues in DNA, particularly cytosine-guanine nucleotides (CpG), can alter gene expression. For example, hypermethylation of CG nucleotides in the promoter regions of tumor suppressor genes diminishes expression of these genes, thereby facilitating the proliferation of colon cancer cells.

Initial epigenetic studies focused on the methylation of DNA in specific genes. More recently developed techniques facilitate the comprehensive genome-wide analyses of the methylation status of DNA in tumors.

Cancer Databases

Extensive data on genomic changes, epigenetic alteration and changes in gene expression in cancer have been compiled by the International Cancer Genome Consortium, ICGC portal https://dcc.icgc.org/ and by the Cancer Genome Atlas (TGCA) cancergenome.nih.gov/.

Analyses of protein changes in cancer are compiled through activities of the Clinical Proteomic Tumor Analysis Consortium CPTAC proteomics. cancer.gov/programs/cptacnetwork.

Specific databases have been established to document somatic mutations in cancer and driver gene mutations e.g. COSMIC cancer.sanger.ac.uk/.

Specific databases have also been developed to document tumor antigens that may be useful in development of vaccines or antibodies to potentially treat tumors e.g. the Cancer Immunome database.

Other important cancer related databases include the therapeutic target database, TARGET (tumor alterations relevant for genomics-driven therapy).

Pavlopoulou et al. (2014) reviewed important tumor related databases.

Circulating Tumor DNA and Liquid Biopsy

There is growing evidence that tumor cells shed DNA into the plasma and into body fluids and that this DNA may be analyzed to assess tumor burden, response to therapy and to detect tumor recurrence.

For analysis of circulating tumor DNA, it is important that the plasma used should be free of white blood cells. Kits are available to amplify DNA through polymerase chain reaction. Sato et al. (2016) emphasized that selected genes tend to be associated with the particular tumor in a patient.

Cell-free circulating DNA analyses are also valuable in analyzing mutations and the mechanisms that lead to development of therapeutic resistance in specific tumors (Meador and Lovly, 2015).

Wang et al. (2015) reported assessment of brain tumors through analysis of cerebrospinal fluid DNA. They reported that if tumors occur adjacent to regions where cerebrospinal fluid circulates, in the brain or in the spinal cord, shed tumor DNA can be identified in cerebrospinal fluid. They determined that assessment of tumor DNA in cerebrospinal fluid can be useful in management of patients with central nervous system tumors.

Exosome Shedding by Tumors

In addition to tumor-derived DNA that is present in plasma, there is evidence that tumors shed small vesicles known as exosomes into blood. Exosomes carry tumor-derived molecules including DNA, mRNA, proteins and other substances from the tumor microenvironment. Exosomes can be purified from plasma and from other body fluids. Components within exosomes may serve as biomarkers for cancer diagnosis (Valencia and Lecanda, 2016).

There is evidence that exosomes derived from tumors that enter blood may also enter distant tissues and carry substances that ultimately facilitate growth of tumor metastases in those organs (Peinado *et al.*, 2011).

A number of investigators have proposed that exosomes may be utilized in the treatment of cancer. Johnsen *et al.* (2014) presented evidence that exosomes may be utilized as drug delivery vehicles.

Emerging Plasma Biomarkers in Cancer Diagnoses

A biomarker is defined as a chemical or biological compound that can be used to diagnose or to monitor disease. One important biomarker is methylated Septin 9 DNA, that has emerged as a biomarker for colon cancer. Methylation of the Septin 9 promoter occurs very frequently in colon cancer tumors (Grutzmann *et al.*, 2008).

More recently, studies on cell-free DNA isolated from plasma have revealed that methylated Septin 9 DNA is an important marker for colon cancer (Molnar *et al.*, 2015).

29 Gene Regulation and "Endless Forms Most Beautiful"

"The uniformity of the earth's life, more astonishing than its diversity, is accountable by the high probability that we derived from a single cell......."

Lewis Thomas (1971) in *The lives of a cell*.

The precise regulation of gene expression that has led to evolution of different life forms and the regulation of processes of differentiation that take place when the fertilized egg develops into an embryo and then into a fetus invoke a sense of wonder.

When I was accepted as a graduate student in human biochemical genetics at University College London, I mentioned to Professor Harry Harris, director of the program, that I was particularly interested in aspects of human genetics relevant to development. Professor Harris agreed that I could undertake studies related to development, provided that they also included an analysis of individual variation (polymorphisms) in proteins.

The best information at that time on differential gene expression of proteins in humans included information on the different types of hemoglobin expression during embryonic, fetal and post-natal life (Huehns et al., 1964). Pikkarainin and Raiha, working in Finland in 1967, described differences in the kinetics of human alcohol dehydrogenase (ADH) in fetal and adult liver. Their study demonstrated that in adult liver the ADH had a pH optimum of 10.4, while ADH in fetal liver had a pH optimum of 10.0. Professor Harris suggested I undertake studies on ADH.

Our studies yielded interesting information on the number of ADH genes and on the expression of the different genes in different tissues and at different stages of development.

As physicians and human geneticists, we eagerly follow new developments and progress in molecular biology and genetics hoping to gain insights that will be useful and help us understand human developmental anomalies and human disease.

Key factors to take into account in considering development and differentiation are firstly, that each nucleus in a particular organism contains all the genes required for development and function of that organism and secondly, that the messenger RNA generated in particular cells in a specific location are specific for that cell type and for that location and for the specific stage of development.

I had a wonderful reminder of how progress in molecular biology, genetics and genomics continues to provide insights into all life on earth when I viewed an amazing series, "What Darwin never knew". Sean Carroll presented wonders of evolution, the diversity, the beauty and the interconnectedness of life forms and brought these into context through information derived from molecular analysis and gene sequencing of different species, different tissues and different life stages.

Interconnected: A Gene Shared Family — the Homeodomain Genes

Homeodomain genes were first studied in the fruit fly *Drosophila*. However, these DNA binding genes occur in many different organisms across the evolutionary spectrum. They are sometimes referred to as body plan genes. Rezsohazy *et al.* (2015) reviewed homeotic genes referred to as Hox genes and their evolution. They reported that invertebrates most frequently have a single Hox gene cluster. In genomes of vertebrates, multiple clusters of Hox genes are present. Hox genes are particularly important for patterning of the axial skeleton.

The Hox genes act as DNA binding factors that impact transcription. In addition, there is evidence that Hox proteins stimulate the assembly of protein complexes. Studies have revealed that Hox proteins impact cell shape, cell proliferation, cell migration, cell differentiation and cell death.

Four clusters of HOX genes occur in the human genome and each cluster contains multiple individual genes. Mutations in at least 10 different HOX genes have been found to lead to specific malformations in humans. These malformations primarily affect skeletal structures, especially long and short bones of limbs. However, the head and face may also be impacted. Specific HOX gene mutations may lead to defects in nails and hair (Quinonez and Innis, 2014).

Temporal and Spatial Differences in Gene Expression at Different Life Stages

Butterflies, birds, reptiles and mammals — in all these groups, studies have revealed that differential gene expression leads to different patterns of coloring and pigmentation. Subtle differences in body forms in a particular species are due to differential gene expression. Oh the wonder of it all!

And then there is the surprising fact; that complexity of life forms does not scale with their gene number.

Following findings from genome sequencing of humans and of many different organisms it has become clear that complexity is not directly related to gene number. Humans have 20,000 genes and the worm *C. elegans* has a similar number of genes.

What makes for increased complexity of form and function?

The key lies in differences in gene regulation and in the capacity of more complex organisms to generate more than one product from each gene.

And so I search more deeply into the unfolding knowledge on regulation of gene expression.

Differences in Expression of Products of a Gene

Developmental biologists currently stress that key factors leading to species differences include the activity of DNA segments they refer to as switches that turn genes on and off at different times and in different tissues. They emphasize, too, that switches are often not located within the specific genes that they impact.

It seems that molecular biologists often favor the term enhancers to describe the genomic segments located outside genes that impact gene expression. Gene expression is then directly dependent on interactions between enhancers and gene promoters.

Enhancers

These are genomic segments located outside of genes and they operate at a distance to impact gene promoters and the initiation of transcription of RNA from protein coding genes. Enhancers differ in size and there is evidence for the existence of enhancer segments. Key elements in enhancers include transcription factor binding sites. Enhancers bind transcription factors that activate them, and there is some evidence that specific factors that bind to enhancers may also inhibit their activation. It appears that several transcription factors on a specific enhancer are required to activate the enhancer and that combinatorial actions of transcription factors are necessary.

Mechanisms by which enhancers impact promoters are being actively investigated. There is evidence that through looping of the strands of chromatin with its embedded DNA, enhancer sequences come to physically interact with promoters. There is also evidence that enhancers produce a specific form of non-protein coding RNA designated as eRNA that interacts with the gene promoter (Anderson et al., 2015). There is also evidence that eRNA derived from enhancers can bind to promoters and impact their activity. The eRNA molecules are non-spliced and non-polyadenylated.

A question that arises is what causes transcription factors to activate enhancers? There is some evidence that specific signaling factors that enter the cell or specific hormonal factors facilitate transcription factor production and enhancer binding (Spitz and Furlong, 2012).

Promoters

Promoters are DNA sequences in the 5' start region of genes that serve to bind and position the enzyme RNA polymerase II adjacent to the transcription start site of the gene and to bind factors that will activate initiation of transcription. Specific sequence elements that may be present in promoters include a TATAAA like elements or a GC box GGGCGGG. These elements are not present in all promoters. The most consistently present sequence element in promoters is CAAT (Strachan and Read, 2010). RNA polymerase II binds to promoter sequence elements through specific proteins often referred to as basal transcription factors, these are TDIIa, TFIIB, TFIID, E, F and I.

Detailed analysis of genes has revealed that many genes have more than one promoter region. Therefore, transcription may be initiated through activity of different promoters and transcripts may be initiated at different transcription start sites. Different promoters and different transcription start sites may be used at different times or in different cell types.

Promoters of genes involved in production of specialized cell proteins are switched off in cells that do not produce that protein; promoters may be turned off through methylation of specific nucleotides, particularly CG dinucleotides. Promoters may be activated when methylation is removed.

Other processes may impact the abundance and the type of product produced by a specific gene. These include selective processing of RNA transcripts, e.g. alternative splicing and generation of different RNA splice forms, differential translation of mRNA that enters the cytoplasm. In addition, different proteins generated during translation may undergo different degrees of cleavage and different secondary modifications.

In an outstanding review of transcription in 2014, Levine, Cattoglio and Tjian wrote:

"We review progress in unraveling one of the outstanding mysteries of modern biology: the dynamic communication of remote enhancers with target promoters in the specification of cellular identity".

In all organisms with DNA in their genome, gene transcription is dependent upon interaction between the RNA synthesizing enzyme RNA polymerase II (POLII) and with sequences in the promoter region at the 5' end of the gene.

Historical concepts of transcription were derived from studies on bacteria (prokaryotes), revealing that specific sequence elements close to the gene promoter played key roles in regulating transcription.

However, differences exist between genes in protozoa and those in higher organisms, Metazoa:

a) Metazoan genes have introns and coding exons. In protozoan genes introns are absent.
b) In metazoan genes, DNA strands are wrapped around nucleosomes which complicates the access of proteins and enzymes to DNA.
c) In metazoans, regulatory sequences can exist in DNA at great distances from the promoter.
d) In vertebrate genes, promoters are impacted by multiple enhancers, including those distant from the promoter. There is evidence that in vertebrates the enhancers may be located more than one megabase distant from the promoter.

Levine *et al.* noted that the location of enhancers at greater distances from a promoter increased possibilities for multiple factors to influence promoter function and likely played roles in increasing diversity of cell types and conditions under which promoters can function and genes can be expressed. The existence of multiple different enhancers located at varying distances from the promoter likely facilitated generation of evolutionary diversity.

The precise mechanisms of communication between enhancers and promoters are still being elucidated.

Insights into Transcription and its Control

Levine *et al.* noted that key factors to consider relevant to the regulation of transcription include histone modification of DNA in the promoter and enhancer regions, specific sequences in enhancers and in promoters and their binding to transcription factors. Levine *et al.* emphasized that 5–10% of the genome in metazoans is involved in encoding transcription factors.

In order to achieve cell type specificity and spatial and temporal differences in gene expression, metazoans utilize multiple and multifaceted promoters and complex machinery for communication between distant enhancers and promoters.

There is evidence that enhancers and core promoters are primed for future activation. One example of such priming presented by Levine *et al.* is that of the FOXA transcription factor, that primes genes in the embryo that are to be expressed in the liver. It has been postulated that priming transcription factors exert their effects through recruitment of histone modifiers or chromatin remodelers.

Levine *et al.* reported that in *Drosophila*, the fruit fly, a specific pioneer transcription factor was shown to mark all genes that would be expressed within 1 ½ to 2 hours after induction of embryogenesis.

There is also evidence that polymerase II is activated through protein binding factors during specific phases.

Levine *et al.* reported evidence that the human genome has larger numbers of enhancers than worms, although the gene numbers are similar in the two. Estimates of the approximate numbers of enhancers in differ-ent organisms were obtained through the ENCODE project. The human genome has approximately 400,000 enhancers, *Drosophila* has between 50,000 and 100,000 enhancers.

Genes are embedded in complex regulatory landscapes sometimes referred to as topological association domains and there is evidence for looping that brings specific domains into contact with each other. In this way, enhancers can be brought into contact with promoters. Deng *et al.* (2012) demonstrated looping between the beta globin promoter regions and its distant regulatory control region.

Villar *et al.* (2015) analyzed enhancers and promoters of genes expressed in the liver of 20 different mammalian species. They reported that there was more rapid evolution of sequences in enhancers than in promoters in higher organisms.

Initiation of promoter activity requires the presence of a pre-initiation complex (PIC) to correctly position polymerase II relative to the transcription initiation site. The pre-initiation complex may contain as many as 12 different subunits. In addition, polymerase requires initiation factors originally referred to as general transcription factors. Coactivators and chromatin remodeling complexes are also required for transcription initiations.

It is important to note that a number of genes have more than one promoter and more than one transcription initiation site. Use of different promoters and transcription initiation sites leads to generation of different transcripts and ultimately to different proteins.

One Gene, Different Transcripts, Different Proteins

Different transcript isoforms may result from use of different transcription initiation sites or from differences in which exons are included in a final transcript. The latter differences result from alternative splicing.

Cell Type Specific Splicing

Zhang *et al.* (2016) reported widespread alternative exon use in specific genes during brain development. They documented in a particular gene that inclusion of a specific exon was different in neuronal precursor cells and in differentiated neurons. Zhang *et al.* determined that in the gene

Ninein a specific exon was removed as neural precursor cells differentiated to neurons. The protein encoded by this gene impacts microtubules.

Another interesting example of alternative splicing and functional effects is the FLNA filamin gene that impacts the cell cytoskeleton. In some transcripts derived from FLNA, an exon that includes a stop codon is included. In FLNA transcripts present in neural progenitor cells this exon is excluded. However, it is included in FLNA mRNA transcripts in neurons in the adult cortex, so that in neurons and adult cortex filamin transcripts are shorter and in fact short transcripts may undergo decay. Zhang *et al.* referred to the specific exon with the stop codon as a "poison exon".

Regulation of Exon Usage

Zhang *et al.* reported that introns that flank exons that are preferentially included in neurons contained specific sequence elements that bound regulatory factors. When the upstream elements bound the PTBP1 RNA binding protein, exon inclusion was suppressed. When RBFOX 1, 2, or 3 RNA binding protein bound to specific downstream intron sequences the specific exon was included.

Zhang *et al.* demonstrated in both mouse and human brains that alternative exon usage plays critical roles in the transition of neuronal precursor cells to neurons.

Hamada *et al.* (2016) demonstrated that the RBFOX family of RNA binding proteins regulate alternate splicing by binding to the specific sequence element: 5'UGCAUGU3' The PTBP1 protein is a polypyrimidine tract binding protein; the polyprotein tract is rich in C and U nucleotides.

Impact of RBFOX1 Gene Expression Levels

Fogel *et al.* (2012) reported that the RBFOX1 RNA binding protein regulates both splicing and more extensive transcriptional networks. In studies on primary human neuro-progenitor cells, they demonstrated that when RBFOX1 was knocked down, significant changes in gene expression resulted. Of particular interest was the fact that RBFOX1 knockdown led to decreased expression of genes required for neurogenesis, neuron development, synaptic transmission and central nervous system development. The list of genes that manifested decreased expression on RBFOX1 knockdown included genes that have been implicated in autism spectrum disorder.

RBFOX1 knockdown in the human neuro-progenitor cells also led to increased expression of certain genes, these included particularly genes involved in metabolic processes.

Regulatory Functions of RNA

For many years the main function of RNA was considered to be related to production of proteins. Messenger RNA transcribed from the gene carries the code for proteins. Transfer RNA and ribosomal RNA utilize the code in mRNA to assemble the amino acid chains of proteins.

In recent decades, however, information has emerged for the existence and function of non-protein coding RNAs. Morris and Mattick (2014) reviewed information on non-protein coding RNAs. Early discoveries of non-protein coding RNA included the small nuclear RNAs (snRNAs) U1–U6 that play important roles in splicing of mRNA and facilitate positioning of the spliceosome.

The snoRNAs are distinct RNAs that are abundant in a nuclear structure referred to as the nucleolus. The nucleolus is involved in the synthesis of ribosomal RNA. SnoRNAs are apparently involved in modification of other forms of RNA, including ribosomal RNA, transfer RNA and snRNAs.

More recently, another form of RNA was identified in a particular nuclear structure known as the Cajal body, spheroid structures that are visible on microscopy of proliferating cells. A form of RNA that accumulates in the Cajal body is designated scaRNA. The scaRNAs are apparently important is generating telomeres at the ends of chromosomes.

Fire, Mello and colleagues reported in 1998 on the occurrence of small double stranded RNAs designated microRNAs. These RNAs interact with sequences at the 3' end of genes and they impact translation of mRNA. MicroRNAs are encoded by genes and are transcribed by RNA polymerase II. The microRNA transcript binds to a specific protein and is transferred to the cytoplasm where it undergoes further processing and protein binding. These processes lead to generation of a complex that impacts the translation of specific target mRNAs on ribosomes.

Another form of small RNAs are designated piRNAs that are expressed primarily in germ cells (particularly in the testis). The piRNAs bind to a specific protein designated Piwi. The piRNA–Piwi protein complex apparently plays a role in suppressing transposable virus-like repeat sequence elements in vertebrate genomes. The piRNA–PIWI complex therefore enhances genome stability in germ cells.

Hombach and Kretz (2016) reported that another form of small RNAs has been identified. These are short double stranded inhibitory RNAs and are referred to as siRNAs.

What Happens to mRNA Spliced out from Introns Contained in Primary RNA Transcripts?

There is growing evidence that the introns that are spliced out from primary mRNA transcripts are repurposed. Hesselberth (2013) reported evidence that spliced out intron-derived transcripts are transported from the nucleus to the cytoplasm. There they likely impact the functions of transfer RNAs and translation of mRNA on ribosomes.

Long Non-coding RNAs

Morris and Mattick (2014) defined long non-coding RNAs as RNAs longer than 200 nucleotides in length that do not encode proteins. Long non-coding (nc) RNAs can be generated from intergenic regions of the genome. Each long ncRNA is transcribed from a specific promoter sequence. Long ncRNAs play important roles in regulation of gene expression. There is also evidence that long ncRNAs influence epigenetic processes. Morris and Mattick proposed that long ncRNAs guide chromatin modifying factors to specific sites.

In addition, many long ncRNAs contain enhancer sequences and are involved in loop formations that bring enhancer sequences in proximity to promoters.

It is important to note that a number of long ncRNAS are transcribed from a promoter close to the 3' end of a gene and generate a transcript that is complimentary to the gene transcript. Binding of the antisense transcript to the original gene transcript will block it and prevent gene expression.

Epigenetics

During the past several decades it has become clear that regulation of gene expression is dependent not only on the nucleotide sequence of

DNA but also on specific modification of the nucleotides. In addition, modifications of histones and alterations in the architecture of the histone-rich chromatin which surrounds DNA play key roles in orchestrating gene expression. In 2016, Allis and Jenuwein documented the history of explorations in epigenetics.

Nucleotide Modifications

Holliday and Pugh (1975) first described modification of nucleotides by methylation. Modification of cytosine by methylation to generate methylcytosine was found to be the most common nucleotide modification. In addition, long stretches of cytosine followed by guanosine were found in the genome and where cytosine was positioned 5' to guanosine, CpG.

These regions were referred to as CpG islands and the extensive methylation of cytosine in CpG islands was found to be associated with suppression of gene expression (Razin and Riggs, 1980; Bird et al., 1985). Specific proteins that bind to methylated DNA were discovered by Meehan et al. (1989).

Chromatin, Histones: Architecture and Modifications

Modifications of histones through addition of acetyl groups was first reported in 1964. Analysis of chromatin by Kornberg in 1974 and microscopic studies by Olins and Olins (1974) delineated the structure of chromatin as repeating units of histones and the occurrence of spherical bodies composed of histones, the nucleosomes. DNA strands were found to be wrapped around the nucleosomes. Nucleosomes were found to be composed of a histone octamer that included two copies each of H2A, H2B, H3 and H4. Nucleosome histones were also found to have tails that projected out from the nucleosome bodies. Strands of DNA between nucleosomes are ensheathed in histones, primarily histone H1.

In 1996, results of intensive studies on histone modifications through methylation and acetylation were reported by Brownell and Allis. Acetylation of histones was found to be associated with activation of gene expression. The enzyme responsible for acetylation was found to be histone acetyl transferase. Subsequently, the enzyme histone deacetylase was found to remove acetyl groups from histones and to inactivate gene expression.

Histones were also found to undergo methylation and this was carried out through activity of the enzyme lysine methyltransferases e.g. KMT2D and KMT2C. Demethylation of histones occurred through activity of histone demethylases e.g. KDM1A.

Jenuwein and Allis (2001) described specific proteins that bind to modified histones and impacted gene expression.

Patterns of Histone Modifications and Gene Expression

Through detailed studies on histone modification and gene expression, epigenetic patterns that impact gene expression were identified. For example, histone H3 lysine 27 trimethylation (H3K27me3) was associated with repression of gene expression. Histone H3 lysine 4 (H3K4me3) was found in actively transcribed genes. Enzymes that modify histones and DNAs have been referred to as writers if they add modifications and they are called erasers if they erase modifications. Histone modification is often insufficient to modify gene expression and binding of additional proteins to modified histones is required (Greer and Shi, 2012). Proteins that bind to modified DNA and histones are referred to as readers. Specific classes of proteins constitute readers.

Chromatin Architecture and Chromatin Remodeling

The spacing of nucleosomes constitutes an important feature of chromatin architecture. Nucleosomes that are close together and tightly packed inhibit binding of transcription factors and other factors that facilitate DNA transcription. Alternatively, DNA transcription is facilitated when nucleosomes are further apart and transcription factors can readily bind to DNA linker strands between nucleosomes and to the histone tails that protrude from nucleosomes. Chromatin remodeling requires energy to alter nucleosome positions.

Transcription Factors

Transcription factors are proteins that contain domains that recognize specific nucleotide sequences in DNA and that bind to these sequences. In addition, many transcription factors contain a second domain that activates transcription. Transcription factors that do not contain this activating domain co-operate with other coactivators to stimulate transcription. Wingender (2013) established a database that documents human transcription factors, TFClass. He reported that there are at least 1,558 different human transcription factors. Through binding to specific sequence elements in gene promoters, in enhancer regions and in silencer regions, transcription factors regulate gene expression.

Nutrition and Epigenetics

Adequate supplies of methyl donors are necessary for the body to carry DNA and histone methylation. The most important methyl donor in the body is S-adenosyl methionine. Synthesis of this metabolite requires B vitamins folate, B_6 and B_{12}.

Environmental Factors and Epigenetics

There is evidence that specific environmental factors can impair epigenetic modification processes. Feil and Fraga (2012) reported evidence that tobacco smoke impacts locus specific methylation, histone modification and chromatin remodeling. Other chemical compounds reported to modify epigenetic processes include asbestos, bisphenol A and benzene.

Deficiencies on our Understanding of Gene Regulation

The fact that four transcription factors can transform differentiated somatic cells into undifferentiated pluripotent stem cells as described by Takahashi and Yamanaka (2006) is still incompletely explained in 2016. Pappetrou (2016) noted that this indicates that some aspects of gene regulation and some functions of transcription factor activity are still unknown.

References

Andersson R, Sandelin A, Danko CG. (2015). A unified architecture of transcriptional regulatory elements. *Trends Genet* **31(8):**426–33. doi: 10.1016/j.tig.2015.05.007. PMID:26073855.

Baltimore D. (1970). RNA-dependent DNA polymerase in virions of RNA tumour viruses. *Nature* **226(5252):**1209–11. PMID:4316300.

Berk AJ, Sharp PA. (1977). Sizing and mapping of early adenovirus mRNAs by gel electrophoresis of S1 endonuclease-digested hybrids. *Cell* **12(3):**721–3. PMID 922889.

Bird A, Taggart M, Frommer M, *et al.* (1985). A fraction of the mouse genome is derived from islands of nonmethylated, CpG-rich DNA. *Cell* **40(1):**91-9. PMID:2981636.

Brenner S, Jacob F, Meselson M. (1961). An unstable intermediate carrying information from genes to ribosomes for protein synthesis. *Nature* **190:**576–581.

Brownell JE, Allis CD. (1996). Special HATs for special occasions: linking histone acetylation to chromatin assembly and gene activation. *Curr Opin Genet Dev* **6(2):**176-84. PMID:8722174.

Carroll S. (2005). *Endless Forms Most Beautiful: The new Science of Evo Devo and the Making of the Animal Kingdom.* Published by W.W. Norton and Company, New York, London.

Caspersson T, Zech L, Johansson C. (1970). Analysis of human metaphase chromosome set by aid of DNA binding fluorescent agents. *Exp Cell Res* **62(2):**490-2. PMID:5495462.

Chow LT, Roberts JM, Lewis JB, Broker TR. (1977). A map of cytoplasmic RNA transcripts from lytic adenovirus type 2, determined by electron microscopy of RNA:DNA hybrids. *Cell* **11(4):**819–36. PMID 890740.

Cirullo RE, Dana S, Wasmuth JJ. (1983). Efficient procedure for transferring specific human genes into Chinese hamster cell mutants: interspecific transfer of the human genes encoding leucyl- and asparaginyl-tRNA synthetases. *Mol Cell Biol* **3(5):**892–902. PMID:6346061.

Crick FH. (1966). The Genetic code. The Croonian Lecture, 1966. *Proc R Soc Lond B Biol Sci* **167(1009):**331–346. (Quotation paragraph 4 introduction, p.331.)

Davidson WM, Smith DR. (1954). A morphological sex difference in the polymorphonuclear neutrophil leucocytes. *Br Med J* **2(4878):**6–7. PMID:13160511.

Deng W, Lee J, Wang H, *et al.* (2012). Controlling long-range genomic interactions at a native locus by targeted tethering of a looping factor. *Cell* **149(6):**1233–44. Doi 10.1016/j.cell.2012.03.051. PMID:22682246.

Dib C, Fauré S, Fizames C, *et al.* (1996). A comprehensive genetic map of the human genome based on 5,264 microsatellites. *Nature* **380(6570):**152–4. PMID: 8600387.

Donahue RP, Bias WB, Renwick JH, McKusick VA. (1968). Probable assignment of the Duffy blood group locus to chromosome 1 in man. *Proc Natl Acad Sci USA* **61(3):**949–55. PMID:5246559.

Doolittle WF, Fraser P, Gerstein MB, *et al.* Sixty years of genome biology. *Genome Biol* **14(4):**113. doi: 10.1186/gb-2013-14-4-113. PMID:23651518.

Doty P, Marmur J, Eigner J, Schildkraut C. (1960). Strand separation and specific recombination in deoxyribonucleic Acids: Physical and Chemical Studies. *Proc Natl Acad Sci USA* **46(4):**461–476.

Duester G, Smith M, Bilanchone V, Hatfield GW. (1986). Molecular analysis of the human class I alcohol dehydrogenase gene family and nucleotide sequence of the gene encoding the beta subunit. *J Biol Chem* **261(5):**2027–33. PMID:2935533.

Feil R, Fraga MF. (2012). Epigenetics and the environment: emerging patterns and implications. *Nat Rev Genet* **13(2):**97–109. doi: 10.1038/nrg3142. PMID:22215131.

Ferguson-Smith MA. (1965). Karyotype-phenotype correlations in gonadal dysgenesis and their bearing on the pathogenesis of malformations. *J Med Genet* **2(2):**142–55. PMID:14295659.

Fire A, Xu S, Montgomery MK, *et al.* (1998). Potent and specific genetic interference by double-stranded RNA in Caenorhabditis elegans. *Nature* **391(6669):** 806–11. PMID:9486653.

Fogel BL, Wexler E, Wahnich A, *et al.* (2012). RBFOX1 regulates both splicing and transcriptional networks in human neuronal development. *Hum Mol Genet* **21(19):**4171–86. doi: 10.1093/hmg/dds240. PMID:22730494.

Friend KK, Dorman BP, Kucherlapati RS, Ruddle FH. (1976). Detection of interspecific translocations in mouse-human hybrids by alkaline Giemsa staining. *Exp Cell Res* **99(1):**31–6. PMID: 57063.

Fu XD, Ares M Jr. (2014). Context-dependent control of alternative splicing by RNA-binding proteins. *Nat Rev Genet* **15(10):**689–701. doi: 10.1038/nrg3778. PMID:25112293.

Gilbert W. (1978). Why genes in pieces? *Nature* **271(5645):**501. PMID:622185.

Graham MA, Barr ML. (1952). A sex difference in the morphology of metabolic nuclei in somatic cells of the cat. *Anat Rec* **112(4):**709–23. PMID:14924252.

Greer EL, Shi Y. (2012). Histone methylation: a dynamic mark in health, disease and inheritance. *Nat Rev Genet* **13(5):**343–57. doi: 10.1038/nrg3173. PMID:22473383.

Grutzmann R, Molnar B Pilarsky C *et al.* (2008). Sensitive detection of colorectal cancer in peripheral blood by septin 9 DNA methylation assay. *PLoS One* **8:**3(11):e3759. doi 10.1371/journal.pone.000375 PMID:19018278.

Gusella JF, Wexler NS, Conneally PM, *et al.* (1983). A polymorphic DNA marker genetically linked to Huntington's disease. *Nature* **306(5940):**234–8. PMID:6316146.

Hamada N, Ito H, Nishijo T, et al. (2016). Essential role of the nuclear isoform of RBFOX1, a candidate gene for autism spectrum disorders, in the brain development. Sci Rep **6**:30805. doi: 10.1038/srep30805. PMID:27481563.

Harper ME, Chan L. (1986). Chromosomal fine mapping of apolipoprotein genes by in situ nucleic acid hybridization to metaphase chromosomes. Methods Enzymol **128**:863–76. PMID:3724532.

Hesselberth JR. (2013). Lives that introns lead after splicing. Wiley Interdiscip Rev RNA **4(6):**677–91. doi: 10.1002/wrna.1187. PMID:23881603.

Holliday R, Pugh JE. (1975). DNA modification mechanisms and gene activity during development. Science **187 (4173):**226-32. PMID 1111098.

Holmes MV, Dale CE, Zuccolo L, et al. (2014). Association between alcohol and cardiovascular disease: mendelian randomisation analysis based on individual participant data. BMJ **349:**g4164. doi: 10.1136/bmj.g4164. PMID:25011450.

Hombach S, Kretz M. (2016). Non-coding RNAs: Classification, Biology and Functioning. Adv Exp Med Biol **937:**3–17. doi: 10.1007/978-3-319-42059-2_1. PMID:27573892.

Hood LE, Hunkapiller MW, Smith LM. (1987). Automated DNA sequencing and analysis of the human genome. Genomics **1(3):**201–12.

Hudson TJ, Stein LD, Gerety SS, et al. (1995). An STS based map of the human genome. Science **270(5244)**: 1945-54. PMID: 8533086.

Huehns ER, Dance N, Beaven GH et al. (1964). Human embryonic hemoglobins. Nature **201:**1095–7. PMID:14152781.

Hurwitz J, Bresler A, Diringer R. (1960). The enzymic incorporation of ribonucleotides into polyribonucleotides and the effect of DNA. Biochem Biophys Res Commun **3:**15–18.

Jenuwein T, Allis CD. (2001). Translating the histone code. Science **293(5532):**1074-80. Review PMID: 11498575.

Keren H, Lev-Maor G, Ast G. (2010). Alternative splicing and evolution: diversification, exon definition and function. Nat Rev Genet **11(5):**345–55. doi: 10.1038/nrg2776. PMID:20376054.

Kornberg A, Lehman IR, Bessman MJ, Simms ES. (1989). Enzymic synthesis of deoxyribonucleic acid. 1956. Biochim Biophys Acta **1000:**57–8. PMID:2673407.

Kornberg RD. (1974). Chromatin structure: a repeating unit of histones and DNA. Science **184(4139):**868-71. PMID: 4825889.

Levine M, Cattoglio C, Tjian R. (2014). Looping back to leap forward: transcription enters a new era. Cell **157(1):**13–25. doi: 10.1016/j.cell.2014.02.009. PMID:24679523.

Leonardo ED, Sedivy JM. (1990). A new vector for cloning large eukaryotic DNA segments in Escherichia coli. Biotechnology (NY) **8(9):**841-4. PMID:1366795.

Lewis SJ, Zuccolo L, Davey Smith G, *et al.* (2012). Fetal alcohol exposure and IQ at age 8: evidence from a population-based birth-cohort study. *PLoS One* **7(11):**e49407. doi: 10.1371/journal.pone.0049407. PMID:23166662.

Lyon MF. (1963). Lyonisation of the X chromosome. *Lancet* **2(7317):**1120–1. PMID:14063435.

Manolio TA. (2013). Bringing genome-wide association findings into clinical use. *Nat Rev Genet* **14(8):**549-58. doi: 10.1038/nrg3523. Review. PMID 23835440.

Maxam AM, Gilbert W. (1992). A new method for sequencing DNA. 1977. *Biotechnology* **24:**99–103. PMID:1422074.

Meador CB, Lovly CM. (2015). Liquid biopsies reveal the dynamic nature of resistance mechanisms in solid tumors. *Nat Med* **21(7):**663–5. doi: 10.1038/nm.3899. PMID:26151324.

Meehan RR, Lewis JD, McKay S, *et al.* (1989). Identification of a mammaliam protein that binds specifically to DNA containing methylated CpGs. *Cell* **58(3):**499-507. PMID:2758464.

Molnar B, Toth K, Bartak BK, Tulassay Z. (2015). Plasma methylated septin 9: a colorectal cancer screening marker. *Expert Rev Mol Diagn* **15(2):**171-84. doi 10.1586/14737159.2015.975212. PMID:25429690.

Morris KV, Mattick JS. (2014). The rise of regulatory RNA. *Nat Rev Genet* **15(6):**423–37. doi: 10.1038/nrg3722. PMID:24776770.

Mullis K, Faloona F, Scharf S, *et al.* (1986). Specific enzymatic amplification of DNA in vitro: the polymerase chain reaction. *Cold Spring Harb Symp Quant Biol* **51(1):**263–73. PMID:3472723.

Nirenberg M, Leder P, Bernfield R, *et al.* (1965). RNA codewords and protein synthesis, VII. On the general nature of the RNA code. *Proc Natl Acad Sci U S A* **53(5):**1161–8.

Ohnesorg T, Vilain E, Sinclair AH. (2014). The genetics of disorders of sex development in humans. *Sex Dev* **8(5):**262–72. doi: 10.1159/000357956. PMID:24504012.

Ohno S, Makino S. (1961). The single-X nature of sex chromatin in man. *Lancet* **1(7168):**78–9. PMID:13730522.

Olins AL, Olins DE. (1974). Spheroid chromatin units (v bodies) *Science* **183(4122):**330-2. PMID:4128918.

Ono M, Harley VR. (2013). Disorders of sex development: new genes, new concepts. *Nat Rev Endocrinol* **9(2):**79–91. doi: 10.1038/nrendo.2012.235. PMID:23296159.

Osier MV, Pakstis AJ, Soodyall H, *et al.* (2002). A global perspective on genetic variation at the ADH genes reveals unusual patterns of linkage disequilibrium and diversity. *Am J Hum Genet* **71(1):**84–99. PMID:12050823.

Ostrer H. (2014). Disorders of sex development (DSDs): an update. *J Clin Endocrinol Metab* **99(5):**1503–9. doi: 10.1210/jc.2013-3690. PMID:24758178.

Papapetrou EP. (2016). Induced pluripotent stem cells, past and future. *Science* **353(6303):** 991–993.

Pavlopoulou A, Spandidos DA, Michalopoulos I. (2015). Human cancer databases (review). *Oncol Rep* **33(1):**3-18. doi: 10.3892/or.2014.3579.PMID:25369839.

Pikkarainen PH, Räihä NC. (1967). Development of alcohol dehydrogenase activity in the human liver. *Pediatr Res* **1(3):**165–8. PMID:6080860.

Pontecorvo G. (1975). Production of mammalian somatic cell hybrids by means of polyethylene glycol treatment. *Somatic Cell Genet* **1(4):**397–400. PMID:1242069.

Quinonez SC, Innis JW. (2014). Human HOX gene disorders. *Mol Genet Metab* **111(1):**4–15. doi: 10.1016/j.ymgme.2013.10.012. PMID:24239177.

Rao VR, Bhaskar LV, Annapurna C, et al. (2007). Single nucleotide polymorphisms in alcohol dehydrogenase genes among some Indian populations. *Am J Hum Biol* **19(3):**338–44. PMID:17421009. DOI:10.1002/ajhb.20589.

Razin A, Riggs AD. (1980). DNA methylation and gene function. *Science* **210(4470):**604-10. PMID: 6254144.

Renwick JH, Lawler SD. (1955). Genetical linkage between the ABO and nail-patella loci. *Ann Hum Genet* **19(4):**312–331.

Rezsohazy R, Saurin AJ, Maurel-Zaffran C, Graba Y. (2015). Cellular and molecular insights into Hox protein action. *Development* **142(7):**1212–27. doi: 10.1242/dev.109785. PMID: 25804734.

Rhoads A, Au KF. (2015). PacBio Sequencing and its Applications. *Genomics Proteomics Bioinformatics* **13(5):**278-89. doi: 10.1016/j.gpb.2015.08.002. PMID:26542840.

Sambrook J, Fritsch EF, Maniatis T. (1989). *Molecular Cloning: A Laboratory Manual*. Cold Spring Harbor Laboratory Press. ISBN 0-87969-309-6.

Sanger F, Nicklen S, Coulson AR. (1977). DNA sequencing with chain-terminating inhibitors. *Proc Natl Acad Sci USA* **74(12):**5463–7. PMID:271968.

Sato KA, Hachiya T, Iwaya T et al. (2016). Individualized mutation detection in circulating tumor DNA for monitoring colorectal tumor burden using a cancer-associated gene sequencing panel. *PLoS One* **11(1):**e0146275. doi: 10.1371/journal.pone.0146275. eCollection 2016. PMID:26727500.

Satre MA, Zgombić-Knight M, Duester G. (1994). The complete structure of human class IV alcohol dehydrogenase (retinol dehydrogenase) determined from the ADH7 gene. *J Biol Chem* **269(22):**15606–12. PMID:8195208.

Seabright M. (1972). Human chromosome banding. *Lancet* **1(7757):**967. PMID:411213.

Search Collaborative Group, Link E, Parish S, et al. (2008) SLCO1b1 variants and statin-induced myopathy – a genomewide study. *N Engl J Med* **359(8):**789-99. doi:10.1056/NEJMoa0801936 PMID:18650507.

Smith DW, Jones KL, Hanson JW. (1976). Perspectives on the cause and frequency of the fetal alcohol syndrome. *Ann N Y Acad Sci* **273**:138–9. PMID:1072342.

Smith HO, Wilcox KW. (1970). A restriction enzyme from Hemophilus influenzae. I. Purification and general properties. *J Mol Biol* **51(2)**:379–391. doi:10.1016/0022-2836(70)90149 X. PMID 5312500.

Smith M, Hopkinson DA, Harris H. (1971). Developmental changes and polymorphism in human alcohol dehydrogenase. *Ann Hum Genet* **34(3)**:251–71. PMID:5548434.

Smith M, Gold P, Shuster J, et al. (1976). Chromosomal assignment of the HL-A common antigenic determinants in man-mouse somatic cell hybrids. *J Immunogenet* **3(2)**:105–15.

Smith M, Hopkinson DA, Harris H. (1971). Developmental changes and polymorphism in human alcohol dehydrogenase *Ann Hum Genet* **34(3)**:251–71. PMID:5548434.

Smith M, Hopkinson DA, Harris H. (1972). Alcohol dehydrogenase isozymes in adult human stomach and liver: evidence for activity of the ADH 3 locus. *Ann Hum Genet* **35(3)**:243–53. PMID:5072686.

Smith M, Hopkinson DA, Harris H. (1973). Studies on the subunit structure and molecular size of the human alcohol dehydrogenase isozymes determined by the different loci, ADH1, ADH2, and ADH3. *Ann Hum Genet* **36(4)**:401–14. PMID:4748759.

Smith M, Hopkinson DA, Harris H. (1973). Studies on the properties of the human alcohol dehydrogenase isozymes determined by the different loci ADH1, ADH2, ADH3. *Ann Hum Genet* **37(1)**:49–67. PMID:4796765.

Smith M, Duester G, Hatfield GW. (1986). Development of DNA probes to investigate genetic variation of alcohol metabolizing enzymes. *NIDA Res Monogr* **66**:50–6. PMID:2883577.

Southern EM (1975). Detection of specific sequences among DNA fragments separated by Gel Electrohoresis. *J Mol Biol* **98(3)**:503–517.

Spitz F, Furlong EE. (2012). Transcription factors: from enhancer binding to developmental control. *Nat Rev Genet* **13(9)**:613–26. doi: 10.1038/nrg3207. PMID:22868264.

Strachan T, Read A. (2010). *Human Molecular Genetics* 4th Edition. Garland Science, p. 14.

Sulem P, Helgason H, Oddson A. et al. (2015). Identification of a large set of rare complete human knockouts. *Nat Genet* **47(5)**:448–52. doi: 10.1038/ng.3243. PMID:25807282.

Takahashi K, Yamanaka S. (2006). Induction of pluripotent stem cells from mouse embryonic and adult fibroblast cultures by defined factors. *Cell* **126(4)**: 663–76. PMID:16904174.

Temin HM, Mizutani S. (1970). RNA-dependent DNA polymerase in virions of Rous sarcoma virus. *Nature* **226(5252):**1211–3. PMID:4316301.

Thomas L. (1971). Notes of a biology-watcher. The lives of a cell. *N Engl J Med* **284(19):**1082-1083. DOI:10.1056/NEJM197105132841908 PMID 5553197.

Valencia K, Lecanda F. (2016). Microvesicles: Isolation, characterization for in vitro and in vivo procedures. *Methods Mol Biol* **1372:**181-92. doi: 10.1007/978-1-4939-3148-4_14.

Villar D, Berthelot C, Aldridge S, *et al.* (2015). Enhancer evolution across 20 mammalian species. *Cell* **160(3):**554–66. doi: 10.1016/j.cell.2015.01.006. PMID:25635462.

Vogelstein B, Papadopoulos N, Velculescu VE, *et al.* (2013). Cancer genome landscapes. *Science* **339(6127):**1546-58, doi:10.1126/science.1235122. Review PMID:23539594.

von Wartburg JP, Schurch PM. (1968). Atypical human liver alcohol dehydrogenase. *Ann N Y Acad Sci* **151(2):**936–46. DOI:10.1111/j.1749-6632.1968. tb48280.x. PMID:4313164.

Wang Y, Springer S, Zhang M, *et al.* (2015). Detection of tumor-derived DNA in cerebrospinal fluid of patients with primary tumors of the brain and spinal cord. *Proc Natl Acad Sci USA* **112(31):**9704–9. doi: 10.1073/pnas.1511694112. PMID:26195750.

Watson JD, Crick FH. (1953). Molecular structure of nucleic acids: a structure for deoxyribose nucleic acid. *Nature* **171:**737–738. doi:10.1038/171737a

Way M, McQuillin A, Saini J, *et al.* (2015). Genetic variants in or near ADH1B and ADH1C affect susceptibility to alcohol dependence in a British and Irish population. *Addict Biol* **20(3):**594–604. doi: 10.1111/adb.12141. PMID:24735490.

Weiss MC, Green H. (1967). Human-mouse hybrid cells containing partial complements of human chromosome and functioning human genes. *Proc Natl Acad Sci USA* **58(3):** 1104-11 PMID: 5233838.

Weiss SB, Gladstone L. (1959). A mammalian system for the incorporation of cytidine triphosphate into ribonucleic acid. *J Am Chem Soc* **81(15):**4118–9. doi: 10.1021/ja01524a087.

Weiss B, Richardson CC. (1967). Enzymatic breakage and joining of deoxyribonucleic acid, I. Repair of single-strand breaks in DNA by an enzyme system from Escherichia coli infected with T4 bacteriophage. *Proc Natl Acad Sci USA* **57(4):**1021–8. PMID: 5340583.

Wilson EB. (1911). The sex chromosomes. *Arch f mikr Anat* **77(1):**249–271. doi: 10.1007/BF02997379.

Wingender E, Schoeps T, Dönitz J. (2013). TFClass: an expandable hierarchical classification of human transcription factors. *Nucleic Acids Res* **41(Database issue):**D165–70. doi: 10.1093/nar/gks1123. PMID:23180794.

Yoshida A, Wang G, Davé V. (1983). Determination of genotypes of human aldehyde dehydrogenase ALDH2 locus. *Am J Hum Genet* **35(6):**1107–16. PMID:6650498.

Zhang X, Chen MH, Wu X, *et al.* (2016). Cell-type-specific alternative splicing governs cell fate in the developing cerebral cortex. *Cell* **166(5):**1147–1162.e15. doi: 10.1016/j.cell.2016.07.025. PMID:27565344.

Zhang Y, Gu N, Miao L, *et al.* (2015). Alcohol dehydrogenase-1B Arg47His polymorphism is associated with head and neck cancer risk in Asian: a meta-analysis. *Tumour Biol* **36(2):**1023–7. doi: 10.1007/s13277-014-2727-x. PMID:25323582.

PART VI

Genetic Variation and Diseases

30 Founder Mutations, Specific Genetic Disorders in Different Countries

In this section I will review evidence that has come to light on the role of specific founder mutations that occur with high frequency in certain populations and likely account for the fact that I encountered more patents with specific disorders in some locations where I worked.

In South Africa, I encountered more patients who had had heart attacks in middle age. Porphyria was a disorder that also occurred more frequently there.

In Scotland, it seemed that hemophilia and cystic fibrosis were relatively frequent in the pediatric population.

In New York at Mount Sinai Hospital, patients with Gaucher disease were frequently seen in clinics and in hospital consultations.

I will revisit these conditions and consider recent molecular genetic studies related to each.

31 Hypercholesterolemia, Heart Disease and Atherosclerosis

In the early 1960s in South Africa, while I participated in collecting blood samples on patients who had had heart attacks to monitor their blood levels of the anticoagulant medication (warfarin) they were prescribed, important information relevant to the cause of coronary heart disease was being gathered in the USA. In 1961, evidence gathered from the Framingham heart study in the USA revealed that abnormal cholesterol levels and high blood pressure were associated with heart disease (www.framinghamheartstudy.org/about-fhs/research-milestones.php).

A key breakthrough in understanding the origins of coronary heart disease was reported in 1979. Goldstein and Brown published evidence that the low-density lipoprotein (LDL) receptor system coordinates the metabolism of cholesterol. In 1983, they published evidence that defects in the low-density lipoprotein receptors (LDLR) played key roles in hypercholesterolemia and atherosclerosis. Goldstein and Brown demonstrated that impaired function of the LDL receptors on the cell surface leads to impaired uptake of cholesterol-loaded lipoproteins into cells. This impaired uptake then triggers increased cellular synthesis of cholesterol. These insights proved to be transformative to the management of coronary heart disease and atherosclerosis.

In 1987, the Food and Drug Administration (FDA) in the USA first approved statins as therapeutic agents for hypercholesterolemia. Statins act as inhibitors of the enzyme HMG co-A reductase; that enzyme is responsible for cellular cholesterol synthesis. In the 1990s, definitive evidence was published that the number of deaths from coronary heart disease and heart attacks was decreased in individuals with hypercholesterolemia who were treated with statins (Tobert, 2003).

In the early 1990s, at the Inborn errors of Metabolism Clinic at UCI, we were consulted about a young female less than 10 years of age that was found to have severely elevated cholesterol levels. The family history in this patient indicated that she likely represented a case of homozygous hypercholesterolemia i.e. she had inherited genes that predisposed to high cholesterol levels and coronary heart disease from both parents. I consulted with other local metabolic specialists and they advised that reducing dietary fat intake was unlikely to significantly impact her cholesterol levels and cardiac disease risk and they had concerns about treating her with statins in view of her young age. Fortunately, we were able refer her to a specialty lipid disease clinic in a nearby city.

During the past two decades much progress has been made in elucidation of factors that cause lipid metabolism impairments and atherosclerosis and more information has been gathered on the genetic factors involved.

Low-density Lipoprotein Receptor (LDLR) Mutations

Studies in different countries have revealed that many different mutations in the LDLR receptor gene on chromosome 19p13.2 can lead to elevated cholesterol levels and to high levels of plasma low-density lipoprotein complexed cholesterol (LDLC). Some patients are true homozygotes in that they inherited identical LDLR gene mutations from each parent. Wiegman et al. (2015) reported that more than 1,700 different LDLR mutations have been reported and that 79% of these likely give rise to a hypercholesterolemia phenotype. In some populations, certain LDLR mutations predominate due to the fact that members of that populations are descendants of a relatively small number of ancestral founders.

The South African Afrikaner population represents an example of a founder population. However, in a study in that founder population of patients with apparently homozygous hypercholesterolemia (based on very high cholesterol levels and family history), Raal et al. (2011) reported that, of 128 patients that had undergone genetic testing, 21 different LDLR mutations occurred; 70 patients were true homozygotes and had inherited the same LDLR mutation from each parent and 58 patients were compound heterozygotes and had inherited a different LDLR mutation from each parent. Raal et al. reported that statin therapy was well tolerated, even by the children with severe hypercholesterolemia who they treated. Raal *et al.* noted that the patients in their study did not achieve the desired level of lowering of cholesterol on statin therapy. Nevertheless, there was evidence that statin therapy delayed adverse cardiovascular events and prolonged patient survival.

Additional Causes of Raised LDL Cholesterol Levels

There is now definite evidence that large effect variants leading to elevated LDL cholesterol levels occur in at least three different genes, namely genes that encode LDL receptor, Apolipoprotein B, and Proprotein convertase subtilisin/kexin type 9 (PCSK9) (Santos *et al.*, 2016). Elevated levels of PCSK9 caused by a specific mutation in the PCSK9 gene lead to accelerated destruction of LDL receptors and to elevated LDL cholesterol. Santos *et al.* emphasized that the different variants in any one particular gene impact cholesterol levels to different degrees.

There is emerging evidence that other genes may also harbor variants that significantly impact cholesterol levels. These include genes that encode Apolipoprotein E, Lipase A, and LDLRAP1, a protein that interacts with the LDL receptor. High plasma levels of Lipoprotein A are also emerging as a risk factor for atherosclerosis.

Specific therapies (inhibitory antibodies) have been developed to treat patients with PCSK9 mutations that predispose to hypercholesterolemia. A molecular therapy has been developed to target a specific damaging mutation in Apolipoprotein B. A drug that limits cholesterol absorption from the small intestine is also used to treat patients who respond poorly to statin therapy.

There is now evidence from large population studies that LDL cholesterol levels in blood are influenced not only by the monogenic gene variants of large effect and by diet, but also by small effect variants in many other genes, referred to as polygenic variants.

Santos *et al.* also emphasized that atherosclerosis is multi-factorial and that there are risk factors other than raised LDL cholesterol levels, these include smoking, diabetes and hypertension.

Cholesterol and lipid levels are, of course, also influenced by diet and levels of physical activity.

32 Cardiomyopathy

In recent decades, studies in South Africa have revealed evidence that heart disease associated with cardiomyopathy (disorders involving the heart muscle) was due to specific mutations that occurred with higher frequency in individuals with the Afrikaner (Dutch) heritage.

Studies on a large North American family and linkage studies led to discovery of genes involved in the etiology of one form of cardiomyopathy, hypertrophic cardiomyopathy. In 1961, Pare reported findings on a large Canadian kindred with a significant family history of heart disease leading to early death. In each of the four generations in this family there were female and male individuals who had been diagnosed with hypertrophic cardiomyopathy. In 1989, Jarcho et al. carried out a genetic linkage study using polymorphic DNA probes to analyze DNA samples from members of the family. At the time of the linkage analysis, 20 affected family members were available for study; 17 of the 20 members had echocardiography results indicative of asymmetric cardiac hypertrophy.

Linkage studies in this kindred revealed that a specific allele of a particular DNA marker D14S26 was found in all affected members. This marker on chromosome 14 mapped in the vicinity of the location of two gene loci, MYH6 and MYH7, that encoded cardiac myosin heavy chains. Subsequent sequence analyses of affected members in this family revealed a missense mutation in exon 13 of the MYH7 gene. This mutation led to a protein change Arg403Glu (Tanigawa et al., 1990).

Additional studies on other families with a history of hypertrophic cardiac myopathy led to the identification of a mutation leading to an Arg453Cys amino acid change.

In 1993, Moolman et al. identified an Arg403Tryp mutation in MYH7 in a South African family with hypertrophic cardiomyopathy.

In 1999, Moolman-Smook *et al.* reported that the MYH7 Arg403Tryp (R403W) variant was embedded in a specific group of variants in a defined genomic segment (a specific haplotype) on chromosome 14, in both the first cardiomyopathy family they reported and in additional South African hypertrophic cardiomyopathy families.

Name of Marker	Allelic Form of Marker
D14S50	7
MYH7 5'UTR	4
MYH 7	403W
MHY6	10
D14S64	3

It is important to note that MYH7 mutations may lead to hypertrophic cardiomyopathy in some patients and to dilated cardiomyopathy in others.

Founder families in South Africa have been found with other mutations that predispose to cardiomyopathies. These include families with mutations in Troponin T, leading to an R92W (Arg92Tryp) amino acid substitution (Moolman-Smook *et al.*, 1999).

Myosin proteins contribute to formation of the cardiac muscle sarcomere structure. Mutations in other genes that encode proteins related to formation of the sarcomere and its connections have subsequently been shown to play roles in cardiomyopathies. Cardiomyopathy-inducing mutations have been identified in myosin heavy and light chain encoding genes, in the MYBPC3 gene that encodes cardiac myosin binding protein C, in cardiac myosin troponins in tropomyosin and in Titin (Lopes and Elliot, 2014).

A founder mutation (2373G) that involved insertion of a nucleotide that disrupted the coding reading frame in the MYBPC3 (myosin binding protein) was also reported to segregate with hypertrophic cardiomyopathy in a family in the Netherlands by Alders *et al.* in 2003.

Watkins *et al.* (2009) reported the occurrence of a specific mutation in Plakophyllin 2 (PKP2) in four different families with Afrikaner heritage. The PKP2 mutation segregated on a specific common haplotype in these families. In these families, the cardiomyopathy was classified as arrhythmo-genic right ventricular cardiomyopathy. Plakophyllins contribute to formation of desmosomes, cytoplasmic structures that are connected to the sarcomere and contribute to cardiac muscle contractile strength.

In a review of gene mutations that play roles in cardiomyopathies, Seidman and Seidman (2011) noted that founder mutations occur more frequently in populations who are more genetically homogeneous, based on geographic or social isolationism. Founder mutations also occur more frequently in a population that suffered earlier calamity so that relatively few individuals survived to produce subsequent generations (population bottlenecks). They also emphasized that mutations may survive in the population if they give rise to conditions that present primarily after middle age years, i.e. after reproductive years.

In studies in a mouse model of the MYH7 mutation p. R403Q (Arg403Glu), Jiang et al. (2013) reported that introduction of an inhibitory RNA to that specific mutation reduced the effect of the mutation. (For more on inhibitory RNA see section on The Future: Molecular therapies).

Hershberger et al. (2013) reported that in 80% of cases of cardiomyo-pathy with genetically based pathogenesis, mutations in MYBPC3 or MYH7 occurred. Furthermore, in 95% of cases of cardiomyopathy with genetic etiology, mutations occurred in one of the following genes: MYBPC3, MYH7, TNNT3 (troponin T3), TNNT2 (troponin T2) or TPM1 (tropomyosin 1).

Hershberger et al. reported that in 50% of cases of genetically determined arrhythmogenic right ventricular cardiomyopathy, desmo-somal proteins were involved – these included DSC2 (desmocollin 2), DSP (desmoplakin) and PKP2 (plakophyllin 2).

Criteria to Determine that a Mutation is Pathogenic

It is important to emphasize that in assigning a specific mutation (a specific sequence variant) as cardiomyopathy-causing it is important that specific criteria be met. These criteria include:

a) Determination that the variant occurs at low frequency in members of the population who do not have the disease.

b) Determining that the specific sequence change is likely to alter the function of the protein encoded by the gene that has the sequence variant. Specific mutations are more likely to be function altering. These include mutations that introduce a stop codon so that translation of the protein is terminated. Insertion of nucleotide(s) or deletion of nucleotide(s) that alter the codon reading frame may lead to production of altered, dysfunctional proteins. Splice site mutations that alter the mRNA transcripts may be damaging. Missense mutations that substitute one amino acid for another may or may not be damaging. In the case of missense mutations, it is helpful to know if the normal amino acid at a particular site is highly conserved across different species. It is also important to consider the position of the change within the protein and if it occurs in important functional domains of the proteins.

c) In evaluating potential pathogenicity of a mutation it is important to carry out searches of the literature and of databases to determine if that specific mutation in the protein has been previously reported in cases with the same disease.

33 Porphyria

As medical students in South Africa, we were taught that Porphyria was a disorder to be considered in the differential diagnosis of adult patients admitted as surgical emergency cases. A professor of surgery reminded us that if a patient presented with abdominal pain, and on examination was found to have multiple abdominal surgical scars from exploratory surgery, we should consider a diagnosis of porphyria and we should order the appropriate clinical chemistry tests. In addition, we were taught that porphyria patients could present with neurological, psychiatric or cutaneous symptoms.

Porphyria was intensely researched and its history in South Africa reported by Geoffrey Dean in 1963.

A Diligent Physician and an Amazing Story

Soon after he settled in South Africa, Dean was consulted about a nurse who had been in an anxious state and took barbiturates. She then developed acute abdominal pain and intestinal obstruction was suspected. Surgery was undertaken with thiopentone (barbiturate) anesthesia; no pathology was found. Two days after surgery she became paralyzed and died. Her urine was reddish brown. Dean spoke to her father: he had ten children and three of his daughters had died with the same symptoms. The father mentioned that he and several of his relatives had sensitive skin that blistered and scarred, "the Van R family skin".

Thus began Dean's investigation of Porphyria Variegata in South Africa. Dean began his study by investigating other descendants of GR Van R (the nurse's great grandfather). Dean writes that when he completed the study, he had traced 434 living descendants of GR Van R and 74 of them had porphyria.

Subsequently, Dean traced descendants of the brothers of GR Van R. The father of these men was then traced in family and church records; he was a GR Van R born in 1768 and his father GR Van R was born in 1732. The brother of the GR Van R born in 1732 had a brother, C Van R, who had sons and daughters, though the daughters had different family names after marriage.

Dean subsequently studied 118 South African family groups with porphyria. He noted that diagnosis of porphyria could be made on the basis of porphyrin studies of urine and particularly through finding excess levels of coprophyrinogen in feces. In severe cases, the presence of this compound could be demonstrated by shining an ultra-violet light (Woods lamp) on the sample.

There was a frequent history of chronic emotional problems and skin problems; however, the acute attacks were usually precipitated by drugs, primarily barbiturates and also sulphonamides.

The important outcome of these studies was that affected individuals were notified about the importance of avoiding specific medications, particularly barbiturates and sulphonamides.

Dean wrote: "In genetic porphyria it is usually the physician who kills the patient, for this reason the possibility of porphyria must always be kept in mind."

It is striking how new therapies lead certain chronic problems to become acute. It is important to note that the list of medications that can precipitate acute porphyria attacks is much longer today than it was during Dean's lifetime.

Porphyria Variegata

The form of porphyria most common in South Africa is variegate porphyria. In addition to neurovisceral symptoms, it is characterized by increased skin sensitivity to sun exposure and increased skin fragility, with tendency to blistering and scarring.

Porphyria variegata is inherited as an autosomal dominant trait: manifestations occur in heterozygotes who carry one copy of the mutant gene. Disease manifestations in heterozygotes usually develop only after puberty. In addition, there is evidence that attacks are precipitated by specific factors including exposure to certain medications, particularly barbiturates. Attacks may also be precipitated by dehydration and by hormonal factors. Attacks occur particularly in women and may be precipitated by altered levels of progesterone and estrogen.

Discovery of the Enzyme Defect in Variegate Porphyria and Characterization of Gene Defect

Brenner and Bloomer (1980) assayed heme biosynthetic pathway enzymes in skin fibroblasts from patients with variegate porphyria and in fibroblasts from unaffected controls. They determined that in patients with variegate porphyria, levels of the enzyme protoporphyrinogen oxidase (PPOX) were significantly reduced compared with levels in controls.

In 1996, the protoporphyrinogen oxidase gene was cloned and sequenced (Dailey and Dailey 1996. In 1996, Meissner, Dailey et al. carried out partial sequencing of the protoporphyrinogen oxidase gene PPOX in South African patients with variegate porphyria and determined that affected patients had a specific mutation that led to an arginine to tryptophan substitution at position 59.

Based on the chromosomal location of PPOX and the gene position of the mutation in cDNA and the variant amino acid the mutation is classified as follows:

1: 61136977, c.175 C>T, R59W (Arg59Tryp) rs 121918324.

Variegate porphyria occurs in individuals in a number of different countries and a number of different gene mutations are responsible. However, the R59W mutation is relatively common in Sweden and in the Netherlands. In 2011, van Tuyll van Serooskerken et al. carried out analyses of 13 polymorphic DNA markers surrounding the site of the R59W mutation in six variegate porphyria patients (three from South Africa and three from the Netherlands) and they reported that there was a core haplotype of seven markers in this region that was identical in the six patients.

Porphyria New York

When I was a junior faculty member at Mount Sinai School of Medicine in New York, I obtained further education on Porphyrias. Dr. Robert Desnick and colleagues carried out research on enzymes involved in porphyrin metabolism. My involvement was to participate in mapping of genes involved in porphyrin metabolism to human chromosomes (Wang et al., 1981).

Dr. Desnick and associates were particularly interested in Acute Intermittent Porphyria (AIP), a condition that has manifestations that overlap in part with the manifestations of variegate porphyria. Both conditions are inherited as autosomal dominant traits and both are associated with acute neurovisceral attacks. In both conditions, the acute attacks require emergency management to ensure adequate hydration, balanced electrolyte status and pain management that does not involve the use of medications that exacerbate the porphyria. Pain medications that include barbiturates are particularly harmful. Acute intermittent porphyria is due to defective function of an enzyme that was initially known as porphobilinogen deaminase, PBGD. Currently this enzyme is referred to as hydroxymethylbilane synthase (HMBS).

In a 2014 review of acute porphyria in the USA, Desnick and collaborators (see Bonkovsky et al., 2014) reported 108 cases of acute porphyria. The report included 90 cases of acute intermittent porphyria with mutations in hydroxymethylbilane synthase, nine cases of variegate porphyria with mutations in protoporphyrinogen oxidase (PPOX) and nine patients who had mutations in coproporphyrinogen oxidase (CPOX).

Clinical histories revealed that all patients had attacks of acute abdominal pain accompanied by evidence of increased sympathetic nervous system activity (hypertension, rapid pulse and sweating). Several of the patients had histories of surgical interventions for similar attacks. The acute attacks often included symptoms of motor weakness, delirium and seizures. Attacks usually commenced between the 2nd and 4th decades of life, and females were affected more frequently than males. Information on factors that precipitate acute attacks of porphyria are available at a number of internet sites, e.g. The European Porphyria Network http://porphyria.eu/.

Some of the patients reported that attacks were less frequent if they had a healthy diet, if they refrained from alcohol consumption and if they engaged in physical exercise.

Bonkovsky et al. (2014) reported that patients having severe attacks responded to treatment with hematin, a medication that is an oxidized component derived from heme.

In acute intermittent porphyria patients in the USA, a range of different hydroxymethylbilane mutations have been found, however the HMBS mutation R116W is apparently more common than other mutations. It is interesting to note that two HMBS mutations occur frequently in Swedish and Dutch patients, HMBS R116W and W198X (where X symbolizes a stop codon mutation). Tjiensvoll *et al.* (2003) reported, however, that the R116W mutation occurred on different haplotypes, indicating that it is likely a recurrent mutation. They reported that the R116W mutation is frequent in acute intermittent porphyria patients in populations in seven different countries: Norway, Sweden, Finland, The Netherlands, France, Spain and South Africa.

34 Gaucher Disease

During my time at Mount Sinai School of Medicine, I also benefited from interactions with clinicians and scientists focused on patient care and research related to Gaucher disease type 1. This disease is also known as non-neuronopathic Gaucher disease. It is an autosomal recessive lysosomal storage disease and affected individuals are most commonly homozygous for a specific mutation. Type 1 Gaucher disease occurs in many different populations, however it is more common in the Ashkenazi Jewish population than in other populations. This disease is due to defects in the function of the enzyme beta glucocerebrosidase (GBA).

In the Ashkenazi population, the mutation in most affected individuals is N370S. Diaz *et al.* (2000) reported that this mutation also occurs in the Spanish and Portuguese populations, however it occurs at much lower frequencies in those populations and homozygotes for the mutation are therefore much less common than in the Ashkenazi population.

At Mount Sinai I was fortunate enough to participate in chromosome mapping of the glucocerebrosidase gene (Shafit-Zagardo *et al.*, 1981).

In recent years, evidence has been gathered which indicates that carriers (heterozygotes) of certain GBA mutations are at increased risk for adult onset Parkinson's disease. This association was first reported by Clark *et al.* in 2007 in the USA population. In 2016, Ran *et al.* reported that in the Swedish population, there was a strong association between risk for Parkinson's disease and specific glucocerebrosidase mutations, particularly GBA L444P and E320K. Individuals heterozygous for either these mutations had an increased incidence of early adult onset of Parkinson's disease compared with the control population. These findings indicate that lysosomal function plays an important role in the pathogenesis of Parkinson's disease.

35 Hemoglobins and Hemoglobinopathies

During our final year of medical school in 1963 a pediatrician presented the case of a young girl who had severe anemia, enlargement of the spleen and thickening of bones of the skull and face. She required frequent blood transfusions. The pediatrician noted that her condition was likely due to impaired regulation of synthesis of hemoglobin. This statement was intriguing but the underlying mechanism was unclear.

The M.Sc. course that I undertook following graduation from medical school and internships provided the opportunity to study genetics, although the lectures included primarily the genetics of plants and of the fruit fly *Drosophila*. I greatly appreciated the assigned textbook by Sinnott, Dobzhansky and Dunn. We used the 1958 edition of that text. In that text the principles of Mendelian genetics and methods used to develop linkage maps of specific phenotypes were clearly described. Discussions on DNA were limited primarily to description of DNA as a component of the nucleus and chromosomes. Evidence that DNA was the transforming principle that led to alterations in the specific types of the pneumococcal bacteria was also discussed. The M.Sc. course also provided opportunities for deeper studies in biochemistry. I was particularly pleased to be instructed to write an essay on hemoglobin. In 1965, I relished the opportunity to delve deeply into the literature on hemoglobin and hemoglobinopathies. Studies of hemoglobinopathies had begun to provide insights into mechanisms through which specific mutations in a protein led to human disease.

As a faculty member at the University of California, Irvine working with the California Newborn Screening program, I again became involved with infants with hemoglobinopathies and their families.

Now, once again, I relish the opportunity to review history and current literature on hemoglobin and related diseases.

History of Hemoglobin and Hemoglobinopathies

There are a number of comprehensive histories on hemoglobin, including those of Edsall in 1972 and a history published by Weatherall, Schechter and Nathan in 2013. David Weatherall also presented interesting aspects of the history of hemoglobinopathies in his book *Science and the Quiet Art*, published in 1995.

Naming of the component that gives blood its red color is attributed to Hoppe-Seyler in 1866. Hoppe-Seyler was a pioneer in the field of physiological chemistry and he established the journal *Zeitschrift fur Physiologische Chemie*. Subsequent work in the late 1800s established that iron was present in hemoglobin, and work in England by Stokes (1852) and others reported changes in the light absorption spectrum of hemoglobin depending on whether or not oxygen was present. The effect of level of acidity (pH) and level of oxygen on the degree of oxygen saturation of hemoglobin was reported by Bohr in Denmark in 1904.

Hemoglobin in Patients with Anemia

Analyses on hemoglobin in patients with anemia are facilitated by the ready availability and easy access to blood. In 1910, Herrick first reported the occurrence of abnormal sickle shaped red blood cells in patients with a severe form of anemia. In 1927, Hahn and Gillespie reported that sickling of red blood cells occurred particularly when oxygen concentrations were low and when deoxyhemoglobin predominated.

Thomas Cooley, a pediatrician, reported in 1925 that severe anemia occurred in children who had enlarged spleens and livers, thickening of the bones of the skull and face and unusual red blood cells. This condition was also known to physicians in Italy. In 1936, Whipple and Bradford assigned the name thalassemia to this condition based on its occurrence in individuals in populations in lands that bordered on the Mediterranean Sea.

Through use of electrophoresis a separation technique developed in 1937 by Tiselius, Pauling *et al.* determined in 1949 that the hemoglobin in patients with sickle cell anemia migrated differently from the normal hemoglobin. In 1949, James Neel, a geneticist, described the inheritance of sickle cell anemia.

In the early 1950s, Vernon Ingram worked on methodologies to enzymatically digest hemoglobin molecules and to derive peptide fragments that could be separated by electrophoresis and chromatography. These techniques led to generation of peptide fingerprints on the separation medium and these could be demonstrated with dyes such as ninhydrin. Peptides could then be eluted and their amino acid sequence could be determined.

In 1956, Ingram reported that a specific peptide, peptide 4, differed in position in sickle hemoglobin as compared with the position occupied by peptide 4 from normal globin. Analysis of the amino acid sequence of the hemoglobin peptide 4 revealed that the peptide fragment unique to sickle hemoglobin varied in its amino acid sequence from the sequence present in normal hemoglobin. In normal globin, the peptide 4 fragment had the amino acid sequence:

Valine-Histidine-Leucine-Threonine-Proline-**Glutamine**-Glutamine-Lysine

Peptide 4 from sickle globin had the amino acid sequence:

Valine-Histidine-Leucine-Threonine-Proline-**Valine** -Glutamine-Lysine

Studies by Rhinesmith, Schroeder and Pauling in 1957 revealed that four different protein N terminals were present in the intact hemoglobin molecule and that this indicated that a hemoglobin molecule was composed of four different subunits. Their studies also revealed that there were two different kinds of subunits in the intact hemoglobin molecule. Two chains were designated as A (alpha) and two chains were designated as B (beta).

In 1958, Smith and Torbert reported results of studies in a particular family in which two different abnormal hemoglobins segregated. In 1959, Ingram and Stretton proposed that different types of hemoglobin defects occurred and that some involved the alpha chain, while others involved the beta chain. Subsequent molecular studies on the family initially described by Smith and Torbert were carried out by Itano and Robinson in 1960. They reported that in some individuals in this family, three different hemoglobins were present. These included two mutant hemoglobins that they labeled HbS and Hb02 and normal hemoglobin HbA. In this family, HbS and Hb02 segregated independently and they concluded that the genes determining them were not linked. Itano and Robinson also demonstrated that HbS and Hb02 mutations were carried on different protein peptides. The HbS mutant was carried on the beta chain and the Hb02 mutant was carried on the alpha globin chain.

In 1959, Ingram and Stretton reported on the genetic basis of thalassemia. They proposed that different types of defects existed in thalassemia, some involved alpha globin defects while others involved beta globin defects. They proposed that the class of mutations that led to non-production of a specific type of globin chain could be caused by a number of different mutations, including deletions, inversions or substitutions. In 1959, Ingram demonstrated that Tiselius electrophoresis of hemoglobins in the presence of an anionic detergent (sodium dodecyl sulfate, SDS) led to separation of the alpha and beta chains of hemoglobin. If the mutation impaired synthesis of a specific globin chain, then that protein could not be detected on electrophoresis of hemoglobin.

In a monograph published in 1961, Ingram emphasized that the study of inherited abnormal hemoglobin in humans revealed the chemical effects of gene actions.

In 1965, Weatherall proposed that an imbalance in the concentrations of alpha and beta chains was the key problem in thalassemias. In beta thalassemias there was impaired synthesis of beta globin chains, and alpha globin chains were present in excess. In alpha thalassemias, where alpha globin synthesis was impaired, beta globins were present in excess. Whenever a specific chain type was present in excess, it precipitated as inclusions in red cells.

In their 2013 review, Weatherall *et al.* wrote:

"By the 1960s and 1970s hemoglobin studies were poised to follow the reconceptualization of biochemistry as molecular biology."

Application of Molecular Biology to the Study of Thalassemias

Methods to isolate messenger RNA from human cells became available in the 1960s (Scherrer *et al.*, 1962). Availability of reverse transcriptase enzymes in the 1970s (Baltimore, 1970) facilitated the generation of cDNA corresponding to globin mRNA from human red cells. In 1972, Ross *et al.* reported *in vitro* synthesis of cDNA complementary to rabbit globin.

Beads attached to oligodeoxythymidine nucleotides (oligo-dT) could be used to isolate messenger RNA that ended in polyadenylation sequences; and in the presence of trinucleotide ATP, GTP, CTP and TTP and reverse transcriptase, cDNA could be synthesized that corresponded in sequence to the mRNA sequence.

In 1976, Maniatis et al. reported isolation of globin cDNA and its cloning into a plasmid. The plasmid was used to transform E. coli. Large amounts of globin DNA could be synthesized from globin cDNA cloned into plasmid or phage vectors.

Labeled cDNA could be used to examine restriction endonuclease digested genomic DNA that had been separated by electrophoresis and adsorbed to nitrocellulose paper.

In addition to sickle cell hemoglobinopathy and thalassemia, many other forms of hemoglobinopathy were identified, particularly in the latter decades of the 20th century.

Intense molecular studies on globins in the 1960s and 1970s revealed that different globin chains were expressed during different life stages, including embryonic, fetal and adult stages. After the neonatal period, adult hemoglobin HbA1 is present, that is composed of two alpha chains and two beta chains ($\alpha2\beta2$). A minor form of hemoglobin present after neonatal life is HbA2 ($\alpha2\delta2$) that is composed of two alpha chains and two delta chains. In early embryonic life alpha globin is not expressed, however an alpha-like globin (the zeta chain) is expressed and epsilon (a beta-like chain) is also produced. In early embryonic life, zeta2 epsilon2 ($\zeta2\ \epsilon2$) is expressed. Subsequently, zeta2 gamma2 ($\zeta2\ \gamma2$) is produced, later in fetal life alpha2 epsilon 2 ($\alpha2\ \epsilon2$) is produced. Towards term and gamma chains are produced and alpha2 gamma2 globin chains combine to produce fetal HbF ($\alpha2\ \gamma2$). Close to the time of birth beta globin chain expression commences and alpha and beta globin chains combine ($\alpha2\ \beta2$).

In 1977, Deisseroth et al. mapped the human alpha globin like gene cluster to chromosome 16. In 1979, the human beta globin gene cluster was mapped to chromosome 11p by Gusella et al.

Linear order of globin loci:

ϵ γG γA δ β beta-like globins on chromosome 11p

ζ α2 α1   alpha-like 16p globins

Thalassemias

"It is under-recognized that what we have learned from the hemoglobin-opathies applies to most human disease and that further analyses of the these uniquely well characterized gene clusters will continue to elucidate important new mechanisms by which mammalian genes are normally switched on and off during cell fate decisions and how this is perturbed in both common and orphan genetic disease". D.R. Higgs (2013).

As noted above, thalassemia syndromes are characterized by reduced output of one or more forms of globin chains. Weatherall and Clegg (1982) reported that a wide variety of different molecular changes lead to defects in globin chain synthesis.

Prior to the elucidation of specific mutations in the beta globin gene, the beta globin thalassemias were often classified as beta thalassemia major or beta thalassemia minor. In beta thalassemia major, beta globin genes on both chromosomes were impacted due (in some cases) to copies of the same mutation being inherited from both parents (recessive inheritance). In some cases, patients with beta thalassemia major were compound heterozygotes; they had inherited two different beta chain mutations, one from each parent. Beta thalassemia major was clinically observed primarily in children and it had defined clinical features. These included failure to thrive, failure to grow normally in weight and height, enlargement of the abdomen due to enlarged spleen, thickening of the skull and facial bones sometimes leading to distortion of the facial features, and reduced body fat.

Enlargement of the spleen leads to trapping of red cells and platelets, this accentuates the shortage of circulating red cells (anemia) and may also lead to shortage of platelets and a tendency to bleed.

Abnormalities of red blood cells are seen microscopically in thalas-semia. These include target cells where pigment appears to be concentrated in the middle of the cell.

In beta0 thalassemia, no beta globin chains are produced; in beta+ thalassemia, small quantities of beta chains are produced. HbA1 ($\alpha2\beta2$) is absent in beta0 thalassemia, however HbA2 ($\alpha2\delta2$) is present in small quantities. Small quantities of fetal hemoglobin ($\alpha2\gamma2$) may be present. Precipitated excess alpha globin chains are particularly present in the red cells in the bone marrow. In heterozygotes who carry one copy of a beta thalassemia mutation, the phenotype varies from completely normal to the presence of anemia.

In rare cases, a mutation in only one of the beta globin genes can lead to beta thalassemia. In such cases, the mutation leads to synthesis of a protein that is extremely unstable.

Molecular defects leading to deficiency of beta globin chains and beta thalassemia include mutations that lead to total deficiency of beta chains and mutations that reduce the quantity of functional beta chains. In some cases, the globin chains are unstable or have impaired function. The majority of beta thalassemia-causing mutations involve one (or a few) nucleotides. Approximately 300 different beta thalassemia-causing mutations are now known (Thein, 2013). These include mutations in the coding region of the beta globin gene and mutations in the 5′ regulatory region of the beta globin gene. The upstream regulatory locus that controls expression of beta globin, LCRB, is located at some distance from the 5′ βglobin transcription start site.

Beta thalassemia-causing mutations have been described in many different population groups. However, this condition occurs primarily in regions of the world where malaria has commonly occurred.

Alpha Thalassemia

Alpha thalassemias occur particularly in regions of the world where malaria has been endemic. In alpha thalassemia, synthesis of alpha globin chains is impaired. The excess beta globin chains form β4 tetramers in post-natal life, referred to as HbH. During fetal life the excess gamma chains form α4 tetramers referred to as HbBarts. HbBarts may lead to abnormal fluid accumulation in the fetus leading to a condition referred to as Hydrops fetalis.

The region on chromosome 16p where the alpha gene cluster is located also contains abundant repetitive DNA elements upstream and downstream of the alpha globin locus. These repetitive elements promote genomic instability and both deletions and duplications of genomic material occurs in this chromosome region. Deletions on chromosome 16p that delete one or more of the alpha globin genes represent common causes of alpha thalassemia. Deletions in 16p may also remove genes that are located close to the alpha globin genes. Very large deletions in chromosomes 16p that remove genes in addition to the globin gene cluster are associated with developmental defects and lead to a syndrome referred to as ATRX syndrome or ATR-16 (Wilkie et al., 1990).

Deletions that remove the alpha1 and the alpha2 globin genes on a specific chromosome may be of different sizes. Two common deletions are the — Sea deletion (deletion of alpha1 and alpha2 from a specific chromosome) and the — Med deletion (deletion of one alpha gene from a specific chromosome). Deletions of a single alpha globin gene on a chromosome may involve the upstream alpha2 gene and have a common size, designated ($-\alpha2^{4.2}$), or the downstream alpha 1 gene ($-\alpha1^{3.7}$).

Non-deletion forms of alpha thalassemia also occur and these are due to mutations that impact regulatory regions or promoter regions of the alpha globin genes. Other disease-causing mutations involve splice sites or result in premature termination of alpha globin gene transcription. In a few cases, deletions of sequences within the alpha globin sequence have been found to cause disease.

Alpha Thalassemia and Clinical Manifestations in World Populations

Vichinsky (2013) reported that alpha thalassemia mutations occur in up to 5% of the world's population. Thalassemia has been reported in all world populations, however it is particularly common in South-East Asia and in parts of China. The frequency is increased in populations of countries that border the Mediterranean Seas.

The term thalassemia major is now used to describe cases that are dependent on blood transfusions for health. The number of alpha genes that are deleted impacts the individual's genotype. Individuals with deletion $-\alpha/\alpha\alpha$ may manifest no symptoms. Individuals with the $-\alpha/-\alpha$ genotype manifest mild symptoms, including anemia. In individuals with $-\alpha/--$ genotype, absence of expression from 3 of the 4 globin genes, beta globin tetramers ($\beta4$) occur and result in hemoglobin H disease. Beta chain tetramers have high oxygen affinity and delivery of oxygen to the tissues is thus impaired.

Non-deletion mutations in the alpha globin gene vary in their effect, and effects are also dependent on whether or not they are co-inherited with alpha gene deletions. One common non-deletion mutant is Hb Constant Spring. This mutation is particularly common in South-East Asian populations. Hemoglobin H disease that occurs in cases that have Hb Constant Spring mutation is associated with severe anemia that follows infections, including viral infections, particularly parvovirus. Patients often manifest severe hemolysis following infections.

Piel and Weatherall (2014) reported that the phenotypic diversity in hemoglobin H disease was wider than originally described and that non-deletion alpha globin variants often caused severe disease. Hemoglobin H disease is characterized by excess beta globin subunits and, in some cases, also by excessive gamma globin subunits.

Hemoglobin H disease may also occur in individuals who have alpha gene deletions ($\alpha/-$, $\alpha/-$), individuals who are compound heterozygotes for globin gene deletions (genotype $\alpha/-$, $-/-$), compound heterozygotes with Constant Spring (cs) mutations ($-/-$, $-/\alpha^{cs}$) and in individuals who are homozygous for Hb Constant Spring mutations (α/α^{cs}, α/α^{cs}). Individuals who are heterozygous for Constant Spring mutations (α/α^{cs}) have few symptoms or mild symptoms. Hb Constant Spring is associated with an elongated alpha gene with 31 extra amino acids.

Vichinsky (2013) emphasized that alpha thalassemia is a major public health problem that requires community support, education and screening in at-risk populations.

Other Hemoglobinopathies that Occur with High Frequencies in Specific Populations

Hemoglobin E (HbE)

HbE is a beta globin structural variant that is synthesized at a slightly reduced rate compared with normal beta globin (Fucharoen and Weatherall, 2012). In HbE homozygotes, there is a mild globin chain imbalance. Minimal abnormalities are present in HbE heterozygotes. In HbE, codon 26 of beta globin is altered and there is a lysine to glutamine substitution. The chain imbalance is likely due to the fact that the HBE nucleotide change also activates a cryptic splice site. The aberrant splicing apparently alters globin processing so that β^E mRNA levels are reduced.

HbE occurs predominantly in South-East Asian populations. Although HbE results in relatively mild changes, when it occurs together with beta thalassemia more significant hematological abnormalities are present. Different phenotypes occur in individuals who are compound heterozygotes for HbE and beta globin mutations that lead to thalassemia. These phenotypes range from mild to more severe anemia.

Hemoglobin C (HbC)

HbC occurs primarily in individuals from West Africa and North-West Africa. HbC is interesting since it involves an amino acid substitution that occurs at the same position as the sickle substitution β6. However, in HbC lysine is substituted for glutamine, whereas in HbS valine is substituted for glutamine at β6. Homozygotes for HbC variants can have mild hemolysis.

My Interest in Hemoglobins Takes a Personal Turn

When I was a graduate student in the PhD program in Biochemical Genetics at University College London (1969–1972), I frequently donated samples of my own blood for experiments that were being carried out by fellow students. Their experiments involved the analysis of enzymes in red blood cells. These enzymes manifested a series of different forms (isozymes) that could be distinguished on starch gel electrophoresis followed by specific staining methods. The stains to detect isozymes contained enzyme-specific substrates and cofactors and dyes. For many of the enzyme systems the specific isozyme pattern observed was influenced by the age of the red cell studied. To confirm the age effect on enzyme patterns, specific separation methods were applied prior to electrophoresis to derive specific populations of young red cells and older red cells. In many experiments, whole blood was used for electrophoresis without prior separation of old and young cells. Students who had used my blood cells in their experiments frequently noted that my whole blood samples manifested isozyme patterns characteristic of young red cells.

Our Professor, Harry Harris, became aware of the finding with my blood and he called me to his office to discuss the results with him. I told him that my bone marrow was likely more active and produced more young cells than normal, since I had a mild hemolytic condition and my bone marrow worked harder to compensate. I told him that my hemolytic condition had been more severe during my early childhood and that my spleen had been removed when I was seven years of age. Following sple-nectomy my health improved greatly. Professor Harris asked me why I had hemolysis and of course the answer was that the cause was not known. I told him that I suspected it was an inherited condition because my mother had an episode of very severe hemolysis at one time in her life, when she was given sulfonamides to treat a bronchial infection.

Professor Harris encouraged me to find out why I had hemolysis and he referred me to a renowned department of hematology at the Hammer-smith Hospital that was located in Shepherd's Bush, a suburb of London. Physicians there discovered that I had an unusual hemoglobin that was initially detected because of its aberrant migration on starch gel electro-phoresis. Further detailed studies on my unusual hemoglobin were carried out in Cambridge, England and its altered amino acid composition was determined. The abnormal hemoglobin was unique and it was designated Hb Shepherd's Bush. At that time, new mutant forms of hemoglobin were given names of the towns where they were discovered. I am heterozygous for this mutation and therefore have one copy of the normal globin gene and one copy of the Shepherd's Bush beta globin gene.

Hb Shepherd's Bush was shown to have an amino acid substitution at position 74 in the βglobin chain, at that position glycine was substituted by aspartic acid. This substitution results in the substitution of a small non-polar amino acid with a large polar amino acid that protruded into the heme pocket of the HbA molecule, and this substitution leads to instability of the hemoglobin molecule. May and Huehns (1972) at University College London subsequently demonstrated that this substitution leads to raised oxygen affinity of HBA and lower reaction with the molecule diphosphoglyc-erate (2-3 DPG). The 2-3 DPG molecule normally acts to promote oxygen release from oxygenated hemoglobin. Destabilization of the abnormal hemoglobin molecule is accentuated under conditions when red cells are stressed by raised temperatures (as during febrile episodes) or when cells are stressed by certain medications.

It is highly likely that my severe hemolytic episodes during child-hood corresponded to periods of childhood illnesses that were likely also treated with sulfonamides, the only antibiotic available during that period (1939–1945). In fact, my mother remembered that doctors frequently pre-scribed M and B tablets to treat throat and ear infections; M and B referred to sulfonamides made and distributed by the pharmaceutical company May and Baker.

Luckily, nurture compensates for nature in our case. My mother and I enjoyed good health if we avoided sulfonamides, had adequate intake of folate and Vitamin B 12 and took care of febrile illnesses promptly.

My Later Involvement with Hemoglobinopathies

In 1981, when I joined the faculty in the Department of Pediatrics at the University of California, Irvine, one of my duties was to provide services related to infants who had been detected on Newborn Screening as having possible inborn errors of metabolism or hemoglobinopathies. The State of California introduced newborn screening for hemoglobinopathies in 1990. Screening was initially for sickle cell disease. However, changes in immigration patterns to California and increased immigration from South-East Asia, particularly after the Vietnam War, and increases in the incidence of clinically significant hemoglobinopathies prompted more comprehensive screening, including screening for HbH disease.

Michlitsch et al. (2009) reported that newborn screening for hemoglobinopathies and follow-up measures decreased mortality in children with sickle cell disease and in children with thalassemia. Specific screening for HbH disease was added to the California Newborn screen based on evidence that children with HbH disease can undergo significant hemolytic episodes during fever and infections, particularly during parvovirus infections. HbH disease can also lead to growth retardation and iron overload. In addition, patients with HbH disease can also undergo bone marrow failure and aplastic crises.

In California, the primary screening of newborns for hemoglobinopathies is carried out by liquid chromatography. Positive cases suspected of having hemoglobinopathy are then referred for confirmatory testing based on electrophoresis and genotyping. Michlitsch et al. reported that in the period between January 1998 and June 2006, confirmed sickle cells disease was observed with a frequency of 1 in 6,600 births, alpha thalassemia occurred with a frequency of 1 in 9,000 births and beta thalassemia occurred with a frequency of 1 in 55,000 births.

Hemoglobinopathies in Europe

In 2014, Suijker *et al.* reported that in the Netherlands the number of children with severe hemoglobinopathies had trebled since 1992. In half of the sickle cell disease patients, their parents originated in West or Central Africa. For children with thalassemia, the majority of parents originated from Morocco or from Asiatic countries.

Aguilar-Martinez *et al.* (2014) reported that major hemoglobinopathies and associated complications were growing problems in Europe due to migration and mobility flows. They noted that target policy measures and action were lacking in the European Union. They recommended that the World Health Organization policies and action measures be followed in the European Union countries.

Current Comprehensive Programs for Treatment of Severe Hemoglobinopathies

Sickle cell disease

McGann *et al.* (2013) reviewed management of cases of sickle cell disease. They emphasized the importance of early detection and the education of parents, families and patients to facilitate early detection of complications. Prophylactic measures include administration of penicillin and pneumococcal immunization. Veno-occlusive episodes must be aggressively treated with administration of fluids, pain medication, antibiotics and transfusion. In addition, screening for evidence of organ damage and stroke are important. Other therapeutic interventions include administration of hydroxyurea and transfusion. In some cases, stem cell transplantation is carried out.

Thalassemias

Olivieri and Brittenham (2013) reviewed management of thalassemias. This includes monitoring of hemoglobin levels in parallel with monitoring of growth and levels of activity to determine when blood transfusions are necessary. Spleen size also needs to be monitored. Assessment of iron levels is important and this includes measurement of ferritin and other iron binding proteins in plasma and assessment of body iron, particularly levels of iron in the liver and heart through magnetic resonance imaging. In some cases, accumulation of excess iron requires chelation therapy.

New Approaches to the Treatment of Beta Globin Hemoglobinopathies

In 2016, Negre *et al.* reviewed new approaches to the treatment of beta hemoglobinopathies. They emphasized that the term thalassemia major is applied now to transfusion-dependent cases of thalassemia irrespective of genotype. Beta thalassemia major results from abnormal beta globin structure or from significantly reduced or absent production of beta chains.

Allogeneic hematopoietic stem cell transplantation is recommended for beta thalassemia major cases. Allogeneic stem cell transplantation is also recommended in young patients with sickle cell disease. However, matched donors are frequently not available.

Clinical trials of gene therapy using the patient's own stem cells are in progress. Other approaches being investigated for beta globin thalassemia and sickle cell disease are methods to enhance production of gamma globin.

Negre *et al.* noted that severe beta thalassemia is frequently associated with one globin gene that is completely silent and with a second globin gene that has the HbE mutation, leading to substitution of the 26th amino acid in the β globin protein glutamine to lysine (Glu26Lys), that leads to abnormal splicing and to transcripts that are poorly translated. In addition, the small quantities of HbE proteins that are produced are very instable.

Investigations into Regulators of Gamma Globin Production

Orkin (2016) reported progress in identification of gene loci involved in the regulation of the switch from gamma globin production to beta globin production. This switch normally occurs in late fetal and early newborn life.

The product of the BCL11A gene was discovered to act as a quantitative regulator of HbF ($\alpha2\gamma2$) production. Other loci important in regulation of the switch are HBS1L and MYB. The globin locus itself also plays a role in switch regulation. However, Orkin emphasized the central role of BCL11A in switch control. He proposes that manipulation of the enhancer of BCL11A expression through gene editing or through methods that inhibit its expression are likely to play important roles in the management of sickle cell anemia and of beta globin hemoglobinopathies in the future.

Pre-clinical Studies Investigating Gene Editing to Treat Hemoglobinopathies

In 2016, there have been a number of interesting reports of pre-clinical use of the CRISPR CAS9 gene editing system to induce gene changes to alleviate hemoglobinopathies. Dever *et al.* (2016) reported correction of the Glu6Val mutation that leads to sickle cell disease. They used patient-derived hematopoietic stem cells and progenitor cells.

Traxler *et al.* (2016) used the CRISPR CAS9 genome editing system to mutate a 13 nucleotide promoter sequence that is present in the gamma1 and gamma 2 globin genes. Editing of these promoters in human erythrocyte progenitor cells caused the gamma globin genes to be continually expressed. Prior clinical studies have revealed that in patients who have mutations that lead to continuous gamma globin production (a condition known as hereditary persistence of fetal hemoglobin), the pathological effects of sickle cell disease and of beta thalassemia inducing mutations are reduced.

36 Hemophilia

The most memorable patient I encountered during the short period in 1966–1967 when I served as a house officer in the medical team at the Children's Hospital in Yorkhill, Glasgow was an approximately three-year-old boy, whom I will call Charlie.

Charlie was brought to the emergency room by his mother on a Saturday afternoon. He had a swollen, inflamed knee that clearly caused him great pain. He also had a slight fever. The emergency room nurse alerted the surgical team, who decided that the joint contained fluid and was likely infected and that surgical drainage was required. Under anesthesia, the surgeon cut into the knee to drain the joint. The surgical incision immediately led to profuse bleeding and it became clear that the joint was filled with fluid blood. It turned out to be very difficult to control the bleeding. The medical team and pathology lab were brought in and the conclusion was reached that Charlie most likely had a defect in coagulation.

Throughout the weekend we worked to monitor Charlie's condition, to replace blood and then to infuse thawed plasma that had been frozen when fresh. Bleeding continued, though less dramatically, over the next few days. The hematologist then had to contact colleagues in London to have plasma cryoprecipitate flown from London to Glasgow. The most likely diagnosis was that Charlie had hemophilia. Studies published in 1965 revealed that cryoprecipitate, a white precipitate formed when plasma is frozen, was much richer as a source of anti-hemophilic proteins than whole plasma.

Charlie's condition improved after the cryoprecipitate infusion. His family was counselled about the ongoing hemophilia management that would be required. It was interesting to note that there was no family history of bleeding disorders.

A few months later, another young child with hemophilia was admitted to our unit. Fortunately, he was less severely affected than Charlie. This five-year-old boy had bumped his head and developed a large hematoma on his forehead. There was no evidence of intra-cranial bleeding. A compression bandage was applied to the forehead and fresh frozen plasma was infused. His condition improved rapidly and in fact it was difficult to keep him from running vigorously around the ward.

These two young boys were my first direct clinical introduction to the bleeding disorder known as hemophilia. The hemophilia story is a fascinating one that includes examples of interesting scientific, clinical and therapeutic breakthroughs and also significant setbacks.

Hemophilia: Breakthroughs and Setbacks

Two types of hemophilia have been identified, A and B. Hemophilia is due to defects in a gene located on Xq28 that encodes a protein known as Factor VIII (FVIII), and hemophilia due to defects in a gene located on Xq27 that encodes a protein known as Factor IX (FIX). Since males have only one X chromosome, defects in the FVIII or FIX lead to hemophilia disease in males. Females have two X chromosomes, so defects in the FVIII or the FIX gene on one X chromosomes are compensated for by the unaffected gene on the second X chromosome. Females may therefore be carriers of hemophilia without manifesting symptoms of the disease. Hemophilia occurs worldwide. The worldwide incidence of hemophilia is estimated to be 1 in 5,000 males and the incidence of hemophilia B is 1 in 30,000 males (Peyvandi et al., 2016).

Hemophilia may present in newborns, particularly in cases where instruments such as forceps or suction were used during delivery. Prolonged bleeding may occur in males with hemophilia who undergo circumcision. Some cases present later as infants and toddlers become more active. Key features include swelling and pain in joints, particularly in ankles, knees and elbows. Repeated bleeding into joints is particularly damaging, leading to long term disability, particularly in cases of severe hemophilia. Bleeding into muscles may also occur. In milder cases of hemophilia, bleeding into joints and tissues may only occur in response to more significant injury. The degree of severity of hemophilia is based on the level of FVIII or FIX in blood. Severe cases have less than 1% of normal values, moderate cases have levels between 1% and 5% of normal and mild cases have between 5% and 40% of normal levels (Kumar and Carcao, 2013).

FVIII acts as a cofactor for FIX. When specific forms of FVIII and FIX combine they serve to activate a complex of FX and FV. In the presence of calcium and phospholipid, the latter complex subsequently leads to the generation of thrombin. Thrombin then converts fibrinogen to fibrin that then forms a clot. Blood clot formation is necessary to stop bleeding.

Treatment of Hemophilia

In the late 1960s, methods were developed to enrich FVIII and FIX from plasma cryoprecipitate. The availability of enriched sources of these factors represented a significant advance in the treatment of hemophilia, since the levels of these protein in whole plasma are very low.

The availability of enriched sources also facilitated isolation of the FVIII and FIX proteins and partial amino acid sequence analysis of the proteins.

In the 1970s, isolation of FVIII and FIX enriched plasma products for treatment of hemophiliacs required collection of batches of plasma from large numbers of donors. By the 1980s it became clear that many batches of plasma carried blood-borne viruses such as HIV and hepatitis, and significant numbers of treated hemophilia patients suffered infection from these viruses. Subsequently, significant efforts were applied to the screening of blood donors and to efforts to neutralize viruses in collected blood.

Isolation, Cloning and Characterization of FVIII and FIX Genes

In November 1984, three remarkable reports appeared in the journal "Nature". Scientists had succeeded in cloning the FVIII gene through screening libraries of genomic and CDNA clones using oligonucleotides corresponding to short segments of the available amino acid sequence of FVIII (Gitschier et al., 1984; Wood et al., 1984; Vehar et al., 1984). They described the complete genomic and exon sequences of FVIII and its amino acid sequence. In addition, they reported that clones containing the FVIII gene could produce FVIII protein.

The human factor VIII gene is a large gene. It spans 186 kilobases, contains 28 exons and it encodes 2,351 amino acids. Gene studies have revealed that at least 2,000 different FVIII mutations occur. Of particular interest was the discovery by Rossiter et al. (1994) of a structural change in the FVIII gene with an internal segment of the gene being flipped over (inverted). Antonarakis et al. (1995) reported that this inversion of intron 22 occurred in 45% of cases with severe hemophilia.

Details of the FIX encoding gene were reported by Lillicrap in 1998. The F1X gene is 34 kb long; it contains eight exons and it encodes 416 amino acids.

Later, an additional hemophilia predisposing inversion in the FVIII gene was identified. This second inversion involves intron 1 and it occurs in approximately 4.8% of patients with hemophilia A, (Cumming, 2004).

Management of Treatment of Hemophilia in Recent Decades

The cloning of the FVIII and the FIX genes led to the availability of these clotting factors through recombinant DNA technology. In addition to increased availability, methods were devised to enhance the half-life of infused FVIII and FIX through specific modification of these proteins.

In addition to the prompt treatment of bleeding and monitoring of joints, programs of preventative therapy were also initiated in several countries. The goal of these programs was to maintain blood levels of the factors at levels that would prevent bleeding through regular infusion of FVIII or FIX in patients with severe hemophilia.

Additional Setbacks: Development of Inhibitors to Infused FVIII or FIX

There is evidence that approximately 30% of patients with severe hemophilia A develop inhibitors to the infused FVIII protein. Development of inhibitors was reported to occur in 4–5% of hemophilia B patients infused with FIX (Peyvandi et al., 2016).

Bypass agents have been developed and are being tested to treat hemophilia patients who have developed inhibitors. One bypass agent is activated prothrombin complex. This complex then permits clotting even if FVIII or FIX are inhibited. Another bypass agent used is recombinant Factor VII that also boosts thrombin formation (Lopez-Fernandez et al., 2016).

Gene Therapy in Hemophilia

Intense efforts have been expended over the past few decades to develop gene therapies for hemophilia. The most successful development has been gene therapy for FIX deficiency, using the FIX gene carried in a specific adenovirus vector, AAV8. On infusion, this adenovirus vector targets the liver. The AAV8 vector was selected since on transfection this vector does not get into the host chromosomes, it exists in the nucleus in an extrachromosomal form (as an episome).

Hemophilia B patients were initially selected for therapy since the FIX gene size makes it more manageable to insert into a vector than the large FVIII gene.

Some success was achieved in gene therapy trials with FIX that were developed and carried out by Nathwani et al. in London (2011). One problem that emerged was that some gene therapy treated patients developed a significant immune response. This was determined to be primarily induced by the capsid (outer shell) proteins in the adenoviral vector. Decrease in immune response was facilitated by ensuring that infused material did not contain free capsid proteins and that the majority of infused capsids contained inserted FIX gene material. Successful gene therapy would eliminate the need for repeated infusion of anti-hemophilic factors throughout the life of hemophilia patients.

An additional important consideration is the high cost of treatments with infused proteins; this is estimated to be greater than 100,000 British pounds per year (Lheriteau et al., 2015).

The Future: Possibilities for Gene Editing in Hemophilia

Early stage clinical trials are in place for gene edited Factor IX. The edited gene has be positioned adjacent to an albumin promoter and this apparently expedites delivery to the liver (https://clinicaltrials.gov/ct2/show/NCT02695160).

37 Cystic Fibrosis

As a house officer involved in the care of newborns at the Queen Mother's Hospital in Glasgow, Scotland in 1967, one of my responsibilities was to work along with the nursing staff to check records and documentation that each newborn had, within the first 48 hours post-partum, satisfactorily passed meconium, the first stool. Meconium contains mucus, degraded cellular materials and bile. Failure to pass meconium could indicate intestinal obstruction in the infant. One form of intestinal obstruction was referred to as meconium ileus and it could be an early manifestation of cystic fibrosis.

A few months later, when I served as a house officer at the Children's Hospital in Yorkhill, Glasgow, I was instructed to perform a sweat test on a young boy who had a history of repeated severe lung infections. At that time, the sweat test was performed by placing a piece of cotton gauze of a defined size on the child's back, covering the gauze with impenetrable plastic and sealing the edges with adhesive tape. The child was then warmly dressed and remained in a warm room. After a set time period the gauze was retrieved and directly placed in a tube that was firmly sealed. This was then sent to the laboratory to check sweat volume and the concentration of chloride present in the sweat. Other important information to be gathered on this child was the nature of his bowel movements and recording of his growth in height and weight since birth. All of this information was important to determine if the diagnosis in this patient was cystic fibrosis.

A History of Cystic Fibrosis

In 1905, Karl Landsteiner (of blood group determination fame) reported a case of intestinal obstruction with thick meconium in an infant who also manifested pancreatic abnormalities. In 1936, Fanconi *et al.* published a report in the German literature documenting the occurrence of a congenital condition associated with abnormalities of the pancreas and disease of the bronchial system. Farber (1944) noted that cystic fibrosis of the pancreas was in fact a multisystem disease and that it was associated with the production of abnormally thick mucus secretions. He proposed that this disease be called mucoviscidosis.

Transformative Reports

Transformative reports on cystic fibrosis appeared in 1951 and 1953. In 1951, Kessler and Anderson documented that, during a severe heat wave in New York, 7 of 12 children who were admitted to the hospital suffering from severe dehydration had cystic fibrosis. The serum chloride levels in these children with cystic fibrosis were found to be abnormally low. In 1953, Di Sant'Agnese *et al.* studied sweat chloride in 43 patients with cystic fibrosis and 50 controls. Sweat collection included application of a dry gauze square of defined size to the back of each child. The gauze was covered with plastic, the edges of the plastic were sealed with adhesive tape, then the children were dressed and placed in a room with temperature at 32°C for 1 to 2 hours. The gauze squares were then placed in stoppered tubes and sent to the laboratory. They determined that the sweat in cystic fibrosis patients contained chloride levels that were, on average, three times higher than those found in controls. These authors also reported that the sweat test results could distinguish patients with cystic fibrosis from patients with celiac disease of the intestine; the sweat test could also distinguish between patients with cystic fibrosis and patients with other chronic lung diseases.

In 1958, Dorothy Anderson published a comprehensive review of the post-mortem pathology-found condition referred to as cystic fibrosis of the pancreas. The exocrine portion of the pancreas was abnormal, with presence of abnormally thick secretions in the pancreatic ducts and distension of the ducts and acini, with the formation of cysts. Abnormal fat infiltration also occurred in the pancreas. She emphasized not only pancreatic abnormalities, but also the respiratory system abnormalities that occurred. These included obstruction of the bronchiole with viscous mucus, dilation of alveoli downstream of obstructed bronchiole, subsequent cyst formation and then collapse of segments of the lung. She also noted that inflammatory changes occurred secondary to bacterial invasion in these patients and that the common organisms that invaded were *Staphylococcus aureus*, *Pseudomonas* and *Proteus vulgaris*. In this series of patient studies, Anderson determined that 10–15% of patients had a history of intestinal obstruction in the newborn period due to meconium ileus. She attributed the abnormally thick meconium to lack of pancreatic digestive enzymes and to abnormal secretions of the intestinal glands.

In 1958, Anderson also reviewed the clinical expressions of cystic fibrosis. She noted that the chronic bronchitis and bronchopneumonia in cystic fibrosis patients could be alleviated to some degree by antibiotic administration. She also reviewed the intestinal problems and celiac disease manifestations that occurred, leading to malabsorption and impaired growth and maturation in cystic fibrosis patients. Deficiency of fat soluble vitamins, particularly vitamin A, also occurred due to poor fat absorption.

Genetics of Cystic Fibrosis

Anderson and Hodges (1946) and Glanzmann (1946) reported that cystic fibrosis of the pancreas was a disease in which genetics played a role. The best proposed model was that it was a recessive disease and that an affected child had inherited a mutant allele from each parent. A parent who carried only one mutant allele did not have manifestations of the disease. By 1961 the term cystic fibrosis of the pancreas became obsolete and the disease name changes to cystic fibrosis (CF).

Eiberg et al. (1985) demonstrated in genetic linkage studies in families that the cystic fibrosis gene mapped to chromosome 7. Tsui et al. (1985) also mapped the cystic fibrosis gene to chromosome 7 through linkage studies. Subsequently, development of additional genetic markers on chromosome 7 and additional linkage studies in families refined more definitively the region on chromosome 7 to which the CF gene mapped. These markers were then used to screen libraries of cloned human DNA to identify a series of overlapping clones. DNA sequencing of the overlapping clones was carried out to identify protein coding segments. Sequencing of DNA from CF patients and controls was then carried out and sequence data was compared to determine if any specific change confined to DNA from CF patients could be identified in protein coding DNA. This strategy was defined as positioning gene cloning.

The finding of a specific 3 base pair deletion in the coding sequence in CF patients signaled identification of the CF gene. This 3 base pair deletion in the coding sequence led to deletion of the amino acid phenylalanine from the CF patient protein. The gene that encoded this protein was designated cystic fibrosis transmembrane conductance regulator (CFTR) and the mutation become known as phe508del (Rommens, 1989). Additional mutations in the CFTR gene were subsequently identified in other CF patients.

In 1991, Drumm et al. analyzed the function of the CFTR gene. They determined that it acted as a chloride conductance regulator. Furthermore, they demonstrated that the phe508del mutation and other CFTR mutations identified in cystic fibrosis patients disrupted chloride conductance.

The CFTR Gene and its Gene Product

CFTR is expressed in epithelial cells in a number of different tissues including lung, pancreas, intestine, liver, gall bladder and sweat glands. It is also expressed at a low level in the kidney and bladder. The CFTR protein forms a channel that is located in the apical membrane of epithelial cells. The CFTR protein produced on ribosomes in the cytoplasm passes to the endoplasmic reticulum, where it must undergo appropriate folding before being transported to the apical membrane of epithelial cells.

The structure of the CFTR protein was reviewed by Ong and Ramsey in 2016. They noted that the CFTR protein has two membrane spanning domains MSD1 and MSD2 that form the channel walls, it also has two intracellular domains and in addition a specific intracellular segment that can be phosphorylated. The function of the CFTR channel is primarily to regulate chloride uptake by the cell. To a lesser extent it also regulates uptake of bicarbonate and other anions. Channel activity is regulated by phosphorylation of the intracellular regulator domain.

CFTR Mutations and their Functional Effects

More than 2,000 different mutations have been identified in CFTR, however, currently only 272 mutations are known to be disease-causing (http:/cftr2.org/). The less common mutations are defined as disease-causing if, along with another known disease-causing mutation, they lead the patient to have an abnormal sweat test with levels of sweat chloride of 60 mmol/L or higher. Another screening test that is used to detect cystic fibrosis is a test to determine whether or not the serum levels of the protein immune reactive trypsinogen are elevated. Elevated levels of immune reactive trypsinogen are indicative of compromised pancreatic function. However, confirmation of cystic fibrosis diagnosis requires a sweat chloride test.

Ong and Ramsey reviewed different types of mutations and their effects on function:

Class 1 mutations produce no protein. These mutations may include stop codon mutations that lead to lack of full length mRNA.

Class II mutations involve changes in the CFTR protein amino acid sequence that prevent correct folding of the protein within the endoplasmic reticulum. Impaired protein folding therefore prevents trafficking to the cell surface.

Class III mutations generate proteins that fail to function appropriately at the cell surface.

Class IV mutations form proteins that form channels, however the channels do not function adequately in chloride conductance.

Class V mutations lead to insufficient protein production.

Class VI mutations lead to proteins with shortened survival time at the cell surface.

Some mutations have more than one effect.

Molecular testing studies of CFTR mutations in a specific patient are important since this information may guide therapy. Ong and Ramsey emphasized that specific types of functional deficiency may need different molecular therapeutic measures in order to be compensated.

In a number of states in the USA, newborn screening is carried out through assessment of levels of immune reactive trypsinogen and in a number of states DNA testing for CFTR mutations and deletions are carried out as part of newborn screening. However, Sosnay et al. (2016) emphasized that the diagnosis of cystic fibrosis is a clinical diagnosis dependent on the results that include quantitative assessment of sweat chlorides.

General Treatment in Cystic Fibrosis

Over the past decades, treatment of CF manifestations has improved the outlook for patients. Available therapies include medications to help promote mucus clearance (mucolytics), physiotherapy, inflatable vests and bronchodilators. Antibiotics specific for the types of invading organisms commonly found in cystic fibrosis patients are also used when infections develop (https://www.cff.org/).

Specific attention has been given to nutrition in cystic fibrosis patients, with addition of pancreatic enzymes, attention paid to vitamin and mineral balance and to adequate sodium chloride intake, especially during warm weather and with increased physical activity.

Molecular Screening for Therapeutic Agents

CFTR variant protein function can be screened in a cellular system. The goal is to carry out high throughput screening with small molecule compounds to determine if any compound restores function of the variant protein.

Ong and Ramsey noted that two classes of small molecule compounds have been distinguished, potentiators and correctors. Potentiators are selected on the basis of their ability to enhance function of proteins that have reached the surface and the goal is to enhance the conductance function of the variant CFTR. Correctors are selected on the basis of their ability to promote transport of the variant to the cell surface by promoting correct folding of the protein.

Based on small molecule screening of CFTR variants, the dug Ivacaftor (Kalydeco) was developed. This drug has been found to improve function of a few different mutations that lead to CFTR conductance defects.

Another drug, Lumacaftor, has been found to improve functions of CFTR variants with abnormal protein folding. One example of such a variant is the CFTR phe508del. Currently (2016) a combination of Ivacaftor and Lumacaftor has US FDA approval for treatment of patients with CFTR phe508del mutations. This is particularly important since phe508del mutations occur in almost 70% of CFTR patients. Another drug, VX-661 is in phase 3 clinical trials for use along with Ivacaftor to treat phe508del mutations, in addition to other specific mutations in class II, III and IV.

Ong and Ramsey noted that class I mutations (due to stop codon mutations) may be partly rescued by drugs such as Ataluren that promote stop codon to read through.

Other Phenotypes that Occur in Patients with CFTR Mutations

Specific mutations in CFTR have been found to occur with higher frequency in individuals prone to sinusitis. In addition, there are specific CFTR mutations that apparently predispose to aberrant development and functions of the vas deferens in males.

38 Inborn Errors of Metabolism

Courses and seminars in biochemistry and metabolism during my student years and later clinical responsibilities led to my education and growing interest in inborn errors of metabolism. Perhaps the most important aspect of these activities was the realization that correct diagnosis of a specific inborn error of metabolism could, in some cases, lead to therapy that would improve the lives of patients.

A First Case

The first patient with whom I was directly involved who turned out to have a treatable inborn error of metabolism was a beautiful infant, Patricia, in the Children's Hospital in Glasgow, Scotland. She was approximately 10 months of age when I first saw her. Patricia was born after a full term pregnancy and normal delivery. Her birthweight and length were average. She breast-fed well during the first three months and her growth was normal. Semi-solid foods were introduced to her diet at about three months. Subsequently, her growth slowed dramatically and at 10 months of age her weight was almost equivalent to her weight at three months of age. Patricia smiled but lay almost motionless in her little crib. Routine clinical testing had failed to reveal a diagnosis and the doctors in our pediatric unit were puzzled and deeply concerned.

One morning, a new doctor attended our ward rounds. He had just returned from visiting clinics in North America. As we stood around Patricia's crib and reviewed her case, the new doctor suggested that she could be a case of hereditary fructose intolerance. He based this suggestion on the fact that Patricia had had normal birthweight, normal growth on breast feeding and the growth defect apparently commenced around the time that semisolid foods were introduced into her diet. Introduced semisolid baby foods often contained sucrose (glucose linked to fructose) and in addition, fruit purees and fruit juices with high fructose content were often introduced at three months. He noted that two tests could be carried out to prove the diagnosis. The first was a fructose tolerance test and the second was a liver biopsy to test for the missing enzyme. Clearly the fructose tolerance seemed to be the best option. I was instructed to carry out the test. Blood samples were to be obtained immediately before fructose administration and at defined intervals after fructose was given. In cases of fructose intolerance, characteristic changes occurred in blood levels of several substances. In typical cases, as blood levels of fructose rose, blood levels of glucose, bicarbonate and phosphorus dropped and levels of blood lactate rose. The patient need to be carefully monitored during the test and if glucose levels dropped too sharply glucose was to be administered.

Results of studies in Patricia confirmed that she did have biochemical manifestations of hereditary fructose intolerance. This disorder was known to be due to deficiency of a liver enzyme, fructose 1-6 biphosphate aldo-lase. All foods that contained fructose were removed from her diet and her subsequent gain in weight and length were really dramatic. As her growth became more normal she began to catch up on developmental milestones.

Patricia's case was, therefore, a wonderful example of the power of correct diagnosis of a problem and of success achieved through initiation of appropriate treatment. Successful treatment of hereditary fructose intolerance was first reported by Black and Simpson in 1967.

Phenylketonuria, Newborn Screening and Inborn Errors of Metabolism Clinic

Experiences in the special clinic for patients diagnosed with phenylketonuria (PKU) provided clear evidence of the importance of early detection and early onset of treatment. Infants detected in early life through the newborn screening program and then placed on a low phenylalanine diet could grow and develop normally. Sadly, in the early days of the clinic we also encoun-tered patients who were born prior to the initiation of newborn screening. Patients with phenylketonuria who were not placed on phenylalanine restricted diets suffered significant developmental delay and cognitive impairment. In addition, they often had troublesome skin conditions.

Advances in the Treatment of PKU

Most cases of PKU are due to mutations in the gene that encodes the enzyme phenylalanine hydroxylase. Detailed studies carried out by Opladen et al. (2012) revealed that in some patients who presented with raised phenylalanine levels, the primary defect was impaired synthesis or function of the tetrahydrobiopterin that is a cofactor for phenylalanine hydroxylase. Initial treatment of PKU was based primarily on reducing phenylalanine content in the diet. In recent years, studies have revealed that addition of tetrahydrobiopterin often increased dietary tolerance of phenylalanine in PKU patients, in patients with phenylalanine hydroxylase mutations. Further advances had included the development of a synthetic form of tetrahydrobiopterin known as Sapropterin. Administration of Sapropterin was reported to permit additional phenylalanine to be added to diets of patients with PKU (Longo et al., 2015).

Advances in Analysis and Treatment of Inborn Errors of Metabolism

During the past half century, many physicians and scientists have worked to elucidate the molecular defects and biochemical pathway defects that lead to inborn errors of metabolism in order to find methods to counteract the consequences of these defects.

Diagnoses of inborn errors of metabolism have been facilitated through expansion of analytical techniques to examine body fluids and in some cases, body tissues. These analytical methods include amino acid analyses and organic acid analyses, through use of chromatography, mass spectrometry and molecular resonance analysis. The goal of these studies is to determine if specific molecules or metabolites are deficient or present in excess amounts and to search for abnormal metabolites.

Other important analytical studies to establish diagnoses include development of assays of enzymes or other proteins to determine if specific qualitative or quantitative changes occurred in patients with specific signs and symptoms.

Over the years it also became possible to analyze specific cellular components and organelles such as lysosomes, mitochondria and peroxisomes. These studies included microscopic analyses and analysis of the functions of the organelles and their specific components.

Newer studies include the use of specific labeled reagents and imaging studies to study accumulation of abnormal components in tissues.

Availability of human genome sequence information and enhanced capabilities to sequence and analyze DNA and RNA have greatly enhanced our capabilities to diagnose genetic diseases, including inborn errors of metabolism (Tarailo-Graovac et al., 2016).

Clinical Presentations of Inborn Errors of Metabolism

Some cases of inborn errors of metabolism may present with acute life threatening illness.

In some cases, impaired growth, developmental delay, or loss of previously attained developmental milestones are the presenting symptoms. In other cases, abnormal organ enlargements, neurological symptoms, or abnormal skeletal findings are the presenting symptoms.

Approaches to the Treatment of Inborn Errors of Metabolism

These include several strategies:

1. Withhold substrates that lead to the accumulation of toxic byproducts in patients with enzyme defects and blocks in metabolism.
2. Attempt to enhance functions of specific enzymes through administration of additional co-factors, e.g. specific vitamins in responsive defects.
3. Provide substances that bind with specific substances that are present in excess and that facilitate the further processing of the excessive substances e.g. administer carnitine to facilitate processing of excessive fatty acids in oxidative disorders.
4. Administer the missing enzyme or protein.
5. If one organ is primarily impacted by the disease, consider organ transplantation.

Lysosomal Storage Diseases

Lysosomes are organelles that contain large numbers of hydrolytic enzymes that are involved in the degradation of complex molecules derived during breakdown of cell membranes and other structures. Lysosomal enzymes function at a low pH and it is therefore important that they be contained within the organelle and separated from the cytoplasm by the lysosome membrane. Deficiencies of specific lysosomal enzymes result in accumulation of undegraded or partially degraded complex molecules within the lysosomes. Lysosomal storage diseases are often classified on the basis of the type of complex macromolecules that accumulate based on deficiencies of specific enzymes.

When I worked as a junior faculty member at Mount Sinai School of Medicine in New York, I had contact with physicians and scientists who carried out pioneering studies on the diagnosis and treatment of two forms of lysosomal storage diseases, Gaucher disease and Fabry disease. In these disorders, the complex molecules stored are defined as glycosphingolipids, containing lipids, complex carbohydrates and ceramide that contains an alcohol group known as sphingosine.

Working in the inborn errors clinic at UCI in California, the lysosomal storage diseases that we most frequently encountered were the mucopolysaccharidoses. These disorders are due to defects in enzymes involved in the breakdown of complex molecules known as mucopolysaccharides (also known as glycosaminoglycans). Different lysosomal enzymes are required for the stepwise degradation of these molecules.

For a number of years, we followed three patients with the Hunter syndrome type of mucopolysaccharidosis that is due to deficiency of an enzyme, iduronate sulfatase, that acts early on in the pathway of mucopolysaccharide degradation. Two of the patients were brothers who suffered from the severe form of Hunters syndrome. These boys both developed signs of the disease when they were between 2 and 3 years of age. These signs included changes in their facial features due to thickening of the soft tissues, joint stiffness, skeletal impairments and progressive cognitive impairments. Both boys died before they reached their teenage years. The third case of Hunter syndrome that we followed was a young man with a milder form of the disorder. Manifestations of Hunter syndrome included increasing skeletal deformities and mobility impairments. He struggled valiantly to lead a normal working life but died in his early thirties.

Over the years, we also followed a young girl with Morquio syndrome (Mucopolysaccharidosis type 3). This disorder results from impaired ability to breakdown the mucopolysaccharide keratin sulfate. This disorder is characterized by impaired growth and skeletal defects.

Another form of storage disease we encountered in two sisters was mucolipidosis. Patients with mucolipidosis have gene mutations that impair the ability of specific enzymes to be correctly targeted to lysosomes. Clinically, patients with mucolipidosis have many of the same problems as patients with mucopolysaccharidoses.

Sadly, for all of the patients mentioned above there was progressive slow deterioration. We could only help by trying to improve mobility, reduce discomfort to some degree and deal with emerging health problems as they arose. We also worked with their families to provide genetic and clinical information and to connect them with support services.

Progress in Enzyme Replacement Therapy

Over the past few decades, extensive efforts have been undertaken to develop therapies for specific lysosomal storage diseases. Major progress has been made in purifying and synthesizing specific lysosomal enzymes that can be used in enzyme replacement therapy. Recombinant DNA techniques have frequently been used to produce the relevant human enzyme in vertebrate cells or in plant cells.

Purified lysosomal enzymes or synthesized recombinant enzymes required to correct the specific enzyme deficiency are administered to patients through intra-venous infusion. The infused replacement enzyme target organs such as liver, kidney, lung, spleen, and heart; however, bone is poorly targeted and the brain is not reached since large molecules do not cross the blood brain barrier. Additional problems related to enzyme replacement therapy include the high cost of therapy and the fact that lifelong treatments are required.

In a review published in 2014, Hollak and Wijburg reported that enzyme replacement therapy had been developed for 19 different lysosomal storage diseases. However, several of these treatments have not been authorized in all countries. Along with efforts to develop new enzyme replacement therapies to target additional lysosomal storage diseases, efforts are continually being applied to identify modifications that will increase the stability of infused enzymes and modifications that will increase patients' immune tolerance of the transfused proteins.

Chaperone Therapy

Other avenues being investigated for treatment of lysosomal storage diseases include development and testing of small molecules known as chaperones that will bind and stabilize lysosomal enzymes. Some of these molecules are closely related to substrates for specific lysosomal enzymes. Hollak and Wijburg reported that galactose was noted to be a chaperone for the alpha galactosidase enzyme that is impacted in Fabry disease. An analog of galactose (1-deoxygalactonojirimycin), also known as Migalastat, has been found to be useful in enhancing activity of alpha galactosidase. In addition, an iminosugar molecule also known as isofagamine, has been shown to enhance activity of the glucosidase enzyme that is defective in Gaucher disease.

Specific molecules have been identified that apparently act by reducing the synthesis of the substrates upon which certain lysosomal enzymes act. The theory is that by reducing synthesis of the substrate in cases with defective lysosomal enzyme activity, a better balance can be achieved between substrate synthesis and substrate degradation. Therapeutic molecules in this category include Miglustat and Eliglustat, investigated for treatment of glycosphingolipid storage disease, and Genistein, an isoflavin molecule purified from soy that apparently decreases synthesis of mucopolysaccharides.

References

Aguilar Martinez P, Angastiniotis M, Eleftheriou A, et al. (2014). Haemoglobino-pathies in Europe: health & migration policy perspectives. *Orphanet J Rare Dis* **9**:97. doi: 10.1186/1750-1172-9-97. PMID:24980780,

Alders M, Jongbloed R, Deelen W, et al. (2003). The 2373insG mutation in the MYBPC3 gene is a founder mutation, which accounts for nearly one-fourth of the HCM cases in the Netherlands. *Eur Heart J* **24(20):**1848–53. PMID:14563344.

Andersen DH, Hodges RG. (1946). Celiac syndrome: V. genetics of cystic fibrosis of the pancreas with a consideration of etiology. *Am J Dis Child* **72(1):** 62–80. PMID: 20994055.

Andersen DH. (1958). Cystic fibrosis of the pancreas. *J Chronic Dis* **7(1)**:58–90. PMID: 13491678.

Antonarakis SE, Rossiter JP, Young M, *et al.* (1995). Factor VIII gene inversions in severe hemophilia A: results of an international consortium study. *Blood* **86(6)**:2206–12. PMID:7662970.

Baltimore D. (1970). RNA-dependent DNA polymerase in virions of RNA tumour viruses. *Nature* **226(5252)**:1209–11. PMID:4316300.

Black JA, Simpson K. (1967). Fructose intolerance. *BMJ* **4(5572)**:138–141.

Bohr C, Hasselbalch K, Krogh A. (1904). Über einen in biologischer Beziehung wichtigen Einfluss, den die Kohlensäurespannung des Blutes auf dessen Sauerstoffbindung übt. *Skand Arch Physiol* **16**:401–412. Translated: Concerning a Biologically Important Relationship: The Influence of the Carbon Dioxide Content of Blood on its Oxygen Binding.

Bonkovsky HL, Maddukuri VC, Yazici C, *et al.* (2014). Acute porphyrias in the USA: features of 108 subjects from porphyrias consortium. *Am J Med* **127(12)**:1233–41. doi: 10.1016/j.amjmed.2014.06.036. PMID: 25016127.

Brenner DA, Bloomer JR. (1980). The enzymatic defect in variegate prophyria. Studies with human cultured skin fibroblasts. *N Engl J Med* **302(14)**:765–9. PMID:7354807.

Clark LN, Ross BM, Wang Y, *et al.* (2007). Mutations in the glucocerebrosidase gene are associated with early-onset Parkinson disease. *Neurology* **69(12)**:1270–7. PMID:17875915.

Cooley TB, Lee P. (1925). A series of cases of anemia with splenomegaly and peculiar bone changes. *Tr Am Pediat Soc* **37**:29.

Cumming AM; UK Haemophilia Centre Doctors' Organization Haemophilia Genetics Laboratory Network. (2004). The factor VIII gene intron 1 inversion mutation: prevalence in severe hemophilia A patients in the UK. *J Thromb Haemost* **2(1)**:205–6. PMID:14717992.

Dailey TA, Dailey HA. (1996). Human protoporphyrinogen oxidase: expression, purification, and characterization of the cloned enzyme. *Protein Sci* **5(1)**: 98–105. PMID 8771201.

Dean G. (1963). The prevalence of the porphyrias. *S Afr J Lab Clin Med* **14**: 145–51. PMID:14110503.

Deisseroth A, Nienhuis A, Lawrence J, *et al.* (1978). Chromosomal localization of human β globin gene on human chromosome 11 in somatic cell hybrids. *Proc Natl Acad Sci USA* **75(3)**:1456–1460. PMID:274732.

Deisseroth A, Velez R, Nienhuis AW. (1976). Hemoglobin synthesis in somatic cell hybrids: independent segregation of the human alpha- and beta-globin genes. *Science* **191(4233)**:1262–4. PMID: 943846.

Deisseroth A, Nienhuis A, Turner P, et al. (1977). Localization of the human alpha-globin structural gene to chromosome 16 in somatic cell hybrids by molecular hybridization assay. Cell **12(1)**:205–18. PMID:561664.

Dever DP, Bak RO, Reinisch A, et al. (2016). CRISPR/Cas9 β-globin gene targeting in human haematopoietic stem cells. Nature **539(7629)**:384–389. doi: 10.1038/nature20134. PMID: 27820943. Doi:10.1038/nature20134.

Diaz GA, Gelb BD, Risch N, et al. (2000). Gaucher disease: the origins of the Ashkenazi Jewish N370S and 84GG acid beta-glucosidase mutations. Am J Hum Genet **66(6)**:1821–32. PMID:10777718.

Di Sant'Agnese P, Darling RC, Perara GA, Shea E. (1953). Abnormal electrolyte composition of sweat in cystic fibrosis of the pancreas. AMA Am J Dis Child **86(5)**:618–9. PMID:13103781.

Drumm ML, Wilkinson DJ, Smit LS, et al. (1991). Chloride conductance expressed by delta F508 and other mutant CFTRs in Xenopus oocytes. Science **254(5039)**:1797–9. PMID:1722350.

Edsall JT. (1972). Blood and hemoglobin: the evolution of knowledge of functional adaptation in a biochemical system. J Hist Biol **5(2)**:205–257. PMID: 11610121.

Eiberg H, Mohr J, Schmiegelow K, et al. (1985). Linkage relationships of paraoxonase (PON) with other markers: indication of PON-cystic fibrosis synteny. Clin genet **28(4)**:265–271.

Fanconi G, Uehlinger E, Knauer C. (1936). Das Coeliakie-syndrom bei angeborener zystischer Pankreasfibromatose und Bronchiektasien. Wien Med Wchnschr **86**:753–756. (Celiac syndrome with congenital cystic fibromatosis of the pancreas and bronchiectasis).

Farber S. (1944). Pancreatic function and disease in early life. V. Pathologic changes associated with pancreatic insufficiency in early life. Arch Pathol **37**:238–250.

Fucharoen S, Weatherall DJ. (2012). The hemoglobin E thalassemias. Cold Spring Harb Perspect Med **2(8)**. pii: a011734. doi: 10.1101/cshperspect.a011734. PMID:22908199.

Gitschier J, Wood WI, Goralka TM, et al. (1984). Characterization of the human factor VIII gene. Nature **312(5992)**:326–30. PMID:6438525.

Goldstein JL, Brown MS. (1979). The LDL receptor locus and the genetics of familial hypercholesterolemia. Annu Rev Genet **13**:259–89. PMID:231932.

Goldstein JL, Kita T, Brown MS. (1983). Defective lipoprotein receptors and atherosclerosis. Lessons from an animal counterpart of familial hypercholesterolemia. N Engl J Med **309(5)**:288–96. PMID:6306464.

Glanzmann E. (1946). Dysporia entero-broncho-pancreatica congenita familiaris. Ann Paediat **166**:289.

Gusella J, Varsanyi-Breiner A, Kao FT, *et al.* (1979). Precise localization of human beta-globin gene complex on chromosome 11. *Proc Natl Acad Sci USA* **76(10):**5239–5242.

Hahn E, Gillespie E. (1927). Sickle cell anemia. *Arch Intern Med* **39:**233–4.

Harris H, Hopkinson DA. (1978). *Handbook of Enzyme Electrophoresis in Human Genetics.* Publishers Elsevier, North Holland Biomedical Press. ISBN 0 7204061.

Higgs DR. (2013). *Hemoglobin and its diseases.* Cold Spring Harbor Laboratory Press. ISBN 0 444 11203 0.

Herrick JB (1910). Peculiar elongated and sickle-shaped red blood corpuscles in a case of severe anemia. *Arch Intern Med (Chic)* **VI (5):**517–521. doi:10.1001/archinte.1910.00050330050003.

Hershberger RE, Hedges DJ, Morales A. (2013). Dilated cardiomyopathy: the complexity of a diverse genetic architecture. *Nat Rev Cardiol* **10(9):**531–47. doi: 10.1038/nrcardio.2013.105. PMID:23900355.

Hollak CE, Wijburg FA. (2014). Treatment of lysosomal storage disorders: successes and challenges. *J Inherit Metab Dis* **37(4):**587–98. doi: 10.1007/s10545–014-9718–3. PMID:24820227.

Hoppe-Seyler. (1866). *Med Chem Untersuch* **1866:**85–116.

Ingram VM. (1956). A specific chemical difference between globins of normal and sickle-cell anemia hemoglobins *Nature* **178(4537):**792–794. doi:10.1038/178792a0. PMID:13369537.

Ingram VM. (1959). Separation of the peptide chains of human globin. *Nature* **27(183):**1795-8.

Ingram VM, Stretton AO. (1959). Genetic basis of the thalassaemia diseases. *Nature* **184:**1903–9 PMID:13852871.

Ingram VM. (1961). *Hemoglobin and its abnormalities.* Charles C Thomas (Publisher), Springfield, Illinois. USA Library of Congress Catalog Card Number: 60–11265.

Itano HA, Robinson EA. (1960). Genetic control of the alpha- and beta- chains of hemoglobin. *Proc Natl Acad Sci USA* **46(11):**1492–501. PMID 16590776.

Jarcho JA, McKenna W, Pare JA, *et al.* (1989). Mapping a gene for familial hypertrophic cardiomyopathy to chromosome 14q1. *N Engl J Med* **321**(20):1372-8. PMID 2811944. DOI:10.1065/NEJM198911163212005.

Jiang J, Wakimoto H, Seidman JG, Seidman CE. (2013). Allele-specific silencing of mutant Myh6 transcripts in mice suppresses hypertrophic cardiomyopathy. *Science* **342(6154):**111–4. doi: 10.1126/science.1236921. PMID:24092743.

Kessler WR, Andersen DH. (1951). Heat prostration in fibrocystic disease of the pancreas and other conditions. *Pediatrics* **8(5):**648–656.

Kumar R, Carcao M. (2013). Inherited abnormalities of coagulation: hemophilia, von Willebrand disease, and beyond. *Pediatr Clin North Am* **60(6):**1419–41. doi: 10.1016/j.pcl.2013.09.002. PMID:24237980.

Landsteiner L. (1905). Darmverschluss durch eingedicktes meconium: pankreatitis. *Zentralbl Allg Pathol* **16**:903.

Lheriteau E, Davidoff AM, Nathwani AC. (2015). Haemophilia gene therapy: progress and challenges. *Blood Rev* **29(5)**:321–8. doi: 10.1016/j.blre.2015.03.002. PMID:26049173.

Lillicrap D. (1998). The molecular basis of haemophilia B. *Haemophilia* **4(4)**:350–7. PMID:9873754.

Longo N, Siriwardena K, Feigenbaum A, *et al*. (2014). Long-term developmental progression in infants and young children taking sapropterin for phenylketonuria: a two-year analysis of safety and efficacy. *Genet Med* **17(5)**:365–73. doi: 10.1038/gim.2014.109. PMID:25232857.

Lopes LR, Elliott PM. (2014). A straightforward guide to the sarcomeric basis of cardiomyopathies. *Heart* **100(24)**:1916–23. doi: 10.1136/heartjnl-2014-305645. PMID:25271316.

López-Fernández MF, Altisent Roca C, Álvarez-Román MT, *et al*. (2016). Spanish Consensus Guidelines on prophylaxis with bypassing agents in patients with haemophilia and inhibitors. *Thromb Haemost* **115(5)**:872–95. doi: 10.1160/TH15-07-0568. PMID:26842562.

Lorkin PA. (1973). Fetal and embryonic haemoglobins. *J Med Genet* **10(1)**:50–64. PMID: 4572642.

Maniatis T, Kee SG, Efstratiadis A, Kafatos FC. (1976). Amplification and characterization of a beta-globin gene synthesized *in vitro*. *Cell* **8(2)**:163–82. PMID:61066.

May A, Huehns ER. (1972). The control of oxygen affinity of red cells with Hb-Shepherds Bush. *Br J Haematol* **22(5)**:599–607. PMID:5032098.

McGann PT, Nero AC, Ware R. (2013). Current management of sickle cell anemia. In: Weatherall D, Schechter AN, Nathan DG (eds). *Hemoglobin and its diseases*. Cold Spring Harbor Laboratory Press, pp. 325–342. ISBN 978-1-936113-45-3.

Meissner PN, Dailey TA, Hift RJ, *et al*. (1996). A R59W mutation in human protoporphyrinogen oxidase results in decreased enzyme activity and is prevalent in South Africans with variegate porphyria. *Nat Genet* **13(1)**:95–7. PMID:8673113.

Michlitsch J, Azimi M, Hoppe C, *et al*. (2009). Newborn screening for hemoglobinopathies in California. *Pediatr Blood Cancer* **52(4)**:486–90. doi: 10.1002/pbc.21883. PMID:19061217.

Moolman JC, Brink PA, Corfield VA. (1993). Identification of a new missense mutation at Arg403, a CpG mutation hotspot, in exon 13 of the beta-myosin heavy chain gene in hypertrophic cardiomyopathy. *Hum Mol Genet* **2(10)**:1731–2. PMID:8268932.

Moolman-Smook JC, De Lange WJ, Bruwer EC, et al. (1999). The origins of hypertrophic cardiomyopathy-causing mutations in two South African subpopulations: a unique profile of both independent and founder events. Am J Hum Genet 65(5):1308–20. PMID:10521296.

Nathwani AC, Tuddenham EG, Rangarajan S, et al. (2011). Adenovirus-associated virus vector-mediated gene transfer in hemophilia B. N Engl J Med 365(25): 2357–65. doi: 10.1056/NEJMoa1108046. PMID:22149959.

Neel JV. (1949). The inheritance of sickle cell anemia. Science 110(2846):64–66. Doi: 10.1126/science.110.2846.64.

Negre O, Eggimann AV, Beuzard Y, et al. (2016). Gene therapy of the β-Hemoglobinopathies by lentiviral transfer of the β(A(T87Q))-globin gene. Hum Gene Ther 27(2):148–65. doi: 10.1089/hum.2016.007. PMID:26886832.

Olivieri NE, Brittenham GM. (2013). Management of the thalassemias. In: Weatherall D, Schechter AN, Nathan DG (eds). Hemoglobin and its Diseases. Cold Spring Harbor Laboratory Press, pp. 271–284. ISBN 978-1-936113-45-3.

Ong T, Ramsey BW. (2016). New therapeutic approaches to modulate and correct cystic fibrosis transmembrane conductance regulator. Pediatr Clin North Am 63(4):751–64. doi: 10.1016/j.pcl.2016.04.006. PMID:27469186.

Opladen T, Hoffmann GF, Blau N. (2012). An international survey of patients with tetrahydrobiopterin deficiencies presenting with hyperphenylalaninaemia. J Inherit Metab Dis 35(6):963–73. doi: 10.1007/s10545-012-9506-x. PMID:22729819.

Orkin SH. (2016). Recent advances in globin research using genome-wide association studies and gene editing. Ann N Y Acad Sci 1368(1):5–10. doi: 10.1111/nyas.13001 PMID:26866328.

Pare JA, Fraser RG, Pirozynski WJ, et al. (1961). Hereditary cardiovascular dysplasia. A form of familial cardiomyopathy. Am J Med 31:37–62. PMID:13732753.

Pauling L, Itano HA, Singer SJ, et al. (1949). Sickle cell anemia, a molecular disease. Science 110:543–548.

Perutz M. (1995). Hoppe-Seyler, Stokes and haemoglobin. Biol Chem Hoppe Seyler 376(8):449–50. PMID:7576244.

Peyvandi F, Garagiola I, Young G. (2016). The past and future of haemophilia: diagnosis, treatments, and its complications. Lancet 388(10040):187–97. doi: 10.1016/S0140-6736(15)01123-X. PMID:26897598.

Piel FB, Weatherall DJ. (2014). The α-thalassemias. N Engl J Med 371(20): 1908–16. doi: 10.1056/NEJMra1404415. PMID:25390741.

Raal FJ, Pilcher GJ, Panz VR, et al. (2011). Reduction in mortality in subjects with homozygous familial hypercholesterolemia associated with advances in lipid-lowering therapy. Circulation 124(20):2202–7. doi: 10.1161/CIRCULATIONAHA.111.042523. PMID:21986285.

Ran C, Brodin L, Forsgren L, *et al.* (2016). Strong association between glucocerebrosidase mutations and Parkinson's disease in Sweden. *Neurobiol Aging* **45**:212. e5–212.e11. doi: 10.1016/j.neurobiolaging.2016.04.022. PMID:27255555.

Rhinesmith HS, Schroeder WA, Pauling L. (1957). A quantitative study of the hydrolysis of human Dinitrophenyl (DNP) globin: the number and kind of polypeptide chains in normal adult hemoglobin. *J Am Chem Soc* **79(17)**: 4682–6. Doi: 10.1021/ja01574a028.

Rommens JM, Iannuzzi MC, Kerem B, *et al.* (1989). Identification of the cystic fibrosis gene: chromosome walking and jumping. *Science* **245(4922)**: 1059–65. PMID:772657.

Ross J, Aviv H, Scolnick E, Leder P. (1972). *In vitro* synthesis of DNA complementary to purified rabbit globin mRNA. *Proc Nat Acad Sci USA* **69(1)**:264–268.

Rossiter JP, Young M, Kimberland ML, *et al.* (1994). Factor VIII gene inversions causing severe hemophilia A originate almost exclusively in male germ cells. *Hum Mol Genet* **3(7)**:1035–9. PMID:7981669.

Santos RD, Gidding SS, Hegele RA, *et al.* (2016). Defining severe familial hypercholesterolaemia and the implications for clinical management: a consensus statement from the International Atherosclerosis Society Severe Familial Hypercholesterolemia Panel. *Lancet Diabetes Endocrinol* **4(10)**: 850–61. pii: S2213-8587(16)30041-9. doi: 10.1016/S2213-8587(16)30041-9. PMID:27246162.

Seidman CE, Seidman JG. (2011). Identifying sarcomere gene mutations in hypertrophic cardiomyopathy: a personal history. *Circ Res* **108(6)**:743–50. doi: 10.1161/CIRCRESAHA.110.223834. PMID:21415408.

Scherrer K, Lathman H, Darnell J. (1962). Demonstration of an unstable RNA and of a precursor to ribosomal RNA in hela cells. *Proc Nat Acad Sci USA* **49**:240–248.

Shafit-Zagardo B, Devine EA, Smith M, *et al.* (1981). Assignment of the gene for acid beta-glucosidase to human chromosome 1. *Am J Hum Genet* **33(4)**: 564–75. PMID 6455062.

Sinnott EW, Dobzhansky T, Dunn LC. (1958). *Principles of genetics, 5th edition.* Published McGraw Hill, N.Y.

Smith EW, Torbert JV. (1958). Study of two abnormal hemoglobins with evidence for a new genetic locus for hemoglobin formation. *Bull Johns Hopkins Hosp* **102(1)**:38–45. PMID:13500096.

Sosnay PR, Raraigh KS, Gibson RL. (2016). Molecular genetics of cystic fibrosis transmembrane conductance regulator: genotype and phenotype. *Pediatr Clin North Am* **63(4)**:585–98. doi: 10.1016/j.pcl.2016.04.002. PMID:27469177.

Stokes GG. (1852). On the change of refrangibility of light. *Phil Trans R Soc Lond* **142**:463–562. doi: 10.1098/rstl.1852.0022.

Suijker MH, Roovers EA, Fijnvandraat CJ, et al. (2014). Haemoglobinopathy in the 21st century: incidence, diagnosis and heel prick screening. Ned Tijdschr Geneeskd **158:**A7365. PMID: 25052352.

Tanigawa G, Jarcho JA, Kass S, et al. (1990). A molecular basis for familial hypertrophic cardiomyopathy: an alpha/beta cardiac myosin heavy chain hybrid gene. Cell **62(5):**991–8. PMID:2144212.

Tarailo-Graovac M, Shyr C, Ross CJ, et al. (2016). Exome sequencing and the management of neurometabolic disorders. N Engl J Med **374(23):**2246–55. doi: 10.1056/NEJMoa1515792. PMID:27276562.

Thein SL. (2013). The molecular basis of β-thalassemia. Cold Spring Harb Perspect Med **3(5):**a011700. doi: 10.1101/cshperspect.a011700. PMID:23637309.

Tiselius A. (1937). A new apparatus for electrophoretic analysis of colloidal mixtures. Trans Faraday Soc **33:**524–531. doi:10.1039/tf9373300524.

Tiselius A. (1968). Reflections from both sides of the counter. Annu Rev Biochem **37:**1–24. doi:10.1146/annurev.bi.37.070168.000245. PMID:4875715.

Tjensvoll K, Bruland O, Floderus Y, et al. (2003-2004). Haplotype analysis of Norwegian and Swedish patinets with acute intermittent porphyria (AIP): Extreme haplotype heterogeneity for the mutation R116W. Dis Markers **19**(1):41-6. PMID 14757946.

Tobert JA. (2003). Lovastatin and beyond: the history of the HMG-CoA reductase inhibitors. Nat Rev Drug Discov **2(7):**517–26. PMID: 12815379.

Traxler EA, Yao Y, Wang YD, et al. (2016). A genome-editing strategy to treat β-hemoglobinopathies that recapitulates a mutation associated with a benign genetic condition. Nat Med **22(9):**987–90. doi: 10.1038/nm.4170. PMID:27525524.

Tsui LC, Buchwald M, Barker D, et al. (1985). Cystic fibrosis locus defined by a genetically linked polymorphic DNA marker. Science **230(4729):**1054–7. PMID:2997931.

van Tuyll van Serooskerken M, de Rooij FW, Edixhoven A, et al. (2011). Digenic inheritance of mutations in the coproporphyrinogen oxidase and protophorphyrinogen oxidase genes in a uniques type of porphyria. J Invest Dermatol **131**(11): 2249-54. doi: 10.1038/jid.2011.186. PMID:21734717.

Vehar GA, Keyt B, Eaton D. (1984). Structure of human factor VIII. Nature **312(5992):**337–42. PMID:6438527.

Vichinsky EP. (2013). Clinical manifestations of α-thalassemia. Cold Spring Harb Perspect Med **3(5):**a011742. doi: 10.1101/cshperspect.a011742. PMID:23543077.

Wang AL, Arredondo-Vega FX, Giampetro PF, Smith M, et al. (1981). Regional assignment of human porphobilinogen deaminase and esterase A4 to chromosome 11q23 leads to 11qter. Proc Nat Acad Sci USA **78**(9): 5734-8. PMID 6946513.

Watkins DA, Hendricks N, Shaboodien G, et al. (2009). Clinical features, survival experience, and profile of plakophylin-2 gene mutations in participants of the arrhythmogenic right ventricular cardiomyopathy registry of South Africa. *Heart Rhythm* **6(11 Suppl):**S10–7. doi: 10.1016/j.hrthm.2009.08.018. PMID:19880068.

Weatherall DJ, Clegg JB. (1982). The molecular genetics of haemoglobin, the thalassaemia syndromes. In: Hardisty RM, Weatherall DJ (eds). *Blood and its disorders, 2nd Edition.* Blackwell Scientific Publications. Chapter 9. ISBN 0-632-00833-4.

Weatherall DJ, Clegg JB, Naughton MA. (1965). Globin synthesis in thalassaemia: an *in vitro* study. *Nature* **208(5015):**1061–5. PMID:5870556.

Weatherall DJ. (1995). *Science and the Quiet Art: The Role of Medical Research in Health Care.* Published by Norton, New York.

Weatherall DJ, Schechter AN, Nathan DG. (eds) (2013). *Hemoglobin and its diseases.* Cold Spring Harbor Laboratory Press. ISBN 978-1-936113-45-3.

Whipple GH, Bradford WL. (1936). Mediterranean disease-thalassemia (Erythroblastic anemia of cooley). *J Pediatr* **9(3):**279–311. Doi: http://dx.doi.org/10.1016/S0022-3476(36)80021-3.

White JM, Brain MC, Lorkin PA, Lehmann H, Smith M. (1970). Mild "unstable haemoglobin haemolytic anaemia" caused by haemoglobin Shepherds Bush(B74(E18) gly--asp). *Nature* **225(5236):**939–41. PMID:5415129.

Wiegman A, Gidding SS, Watts GF, et al. (2015). Familial hypercholesterolaemia in children and adolescents: gaining decades of life by optimizing detection and treatment. *Eur Heart J* **36(36):**2425–37. doi: 10.1093/eurheartj/ehv157. PMID:26009596.

Wilkie AO, Buckle VJ, Harris PC, et al. (1990). Clinical features and molecular analysis of the alpha thalassemia/mental retardation syndromes. I. Cases due to deletions involving chromosome band 16p13.3. *Am J Hum Genet* **46(6):**1112–26. PMID:233970.

Wood WI, Capon DJ, Simonsen CC, et al. (1984). Expression of active human factor VIII from recombinant DNA clones. *Nature* **312(5992):**330–7. PMID:6438526.

PART VII

Complexities and Striving for Insights

39 Evolution of Therapies, Complexities, Root Causes, and Moves Toward Personalized Medicine

Therapies in Modern Times

A brief outline of therapeutic approaches in modern times could include the following topics:

1. Management of symptoms.
2. Removal of damaging or disruptive lesions.
3. Use of specific therapeutic agents or specific measures based on determination of the root cause of the disease.
4. Prevention measures based on understanding of causative factors, e.g. micro-organisms, diet, environmental factors.
5. Use of therapeutic agents, therapeutic measures, or symptom relieving measures based on evidence gathered from large population studies.
6. Use of therapeutic agents, therapeutic measures, or symptom relieving measures taking into account specific attributes of the patient, including genetic factors, life factors and life choice.

Addressing Root Causes

Discoveries of root causes of specific diseases have been among the great achievements of the late 19th and the 20th century. Early examples included the discovery of microorganisms and their roles in infectious disease, discovery of vitamins and recognition of manifestations of their deficiency, and discovery of antibiotics.

Moving further into the 20th century, discovery of the root causes of diabetes, coronary heart diseases, atherosclerosis and of immunologically determined diseases, and development of therapeutic measures were triumphs.

Lewis Thomas celebrated the optimism engendered by some of these achievements in several of his remarkable essays. He particularly drew attention to the important role of basic research in laying the groundwork for clinical advances.

In 1974, Thomas wrote:

"There is an abundance of interesting facts relating to all our major diseases and more items of information are coming in steadily from all quarters of biology".

Thomas also wrote of medicine and therapeutics in terms of technologies. He defined firstly "non-technology", for example, supportive care. "It tides patients through diseases that are not understood". He realized that this was valued by patients. He noted that it required much professional time and he thought it contributed substantially to healthcare expenses.

Thomas then defined a category which he designated "halfway technology", used to compensate for the incapacitating effects of certain diseases that were only managed at late stages: "Diseases that one is not able to do very much about". Examples of halfway technology that Thomas presented included the use of dialysis and transplants for kidneys damaged by poorly understood diseases. He considered the extensive expenses of sophisticated units to manage myocardial infarction and heart transplants as examples of halfway technology. Thomas proposed: "The real high technology of medicine comes as the result of a genuine understanding of disease mechanisms".

I celebrate Lewis Thomas' insights, his erudition and his enthusiasm. There are indeed many examples of diseases where understanding of the basic disease mechanism has led to introduction of revolutionary therapies. In the area of genetic diseases, understanding of specific disease mechanisms of inborn errors of metabolism, for example pathogenesis of phenylketonuria, led to implementation of modified diets that prevented damaging effects of accumulated toxic metabolites and prevention of post-natal brain damage. Other more recent examples include the discovery of specific gene mutations through sequencing analysis and design of therapies to bypass or mitigate the effects of the gene defect. In one recent example, discovery of gene defects in enzymes involved in catecholamine and dopamine-related synthesis and metabolism led to implementation of specific therapies that relieved severe neurological symptoms and spasticity (Bainbridge et al., 2011).

Complex Causation

Complexities of causation, particularly in common diseases, are dependent not only on gene–environment interactions, but also on additive effects of variants in numbers of different genes relevant to the functioning of particular biological systems. In addition, interactions between genes (epistatic effects) may have effects. Hall et al. (2016) noted that interactive gene effects are quite difficult to clearly demonstrate using current statistical methods.

More comprehensive analysis methods are currently being developed to analyze the effects of environmental effects on disease causation, referred to as EWAS. In addition, sophisticated analysis methods are required to analyze gene–environment interactions (Hall et al., 2016).

Genome-wide Association Studies (GWAS)

Comprehensive genome-wide association studies have been carried out over the past several decades to provide insight into gene variants that impact common diseases, including diabetes, cardiovascular disease and metabolic diseases. When very large number of individuals in a population were studied and when studies included affected individuals and unaffected controls, statistically significant genotype disease associations were sometimes obtained. However, in the majority of cases, the genetic variants found only slightly altered the risk of determining disease. For example, in statistically significant studies the odds ratio of developing a disease when the risk allele was present were most commonly 1.2 to 1.4 (Hall et al., 2016). The OR represents the odds that an outcome (e.g. a particular disease) will occur given a particular exposure, compared to the odds of the outcome occurring in the absence of that exposure.

Gene–Environment Interactions and Natural Selection

There is evidence that specific environmental factors, including dietary factors, elevation above sea level and exposure to specific parasites influence the selection of specific genetic variants (DNA nucleotides), and therefore influence the frequency of specific genetic variants in populations living in different parts of the world.

Specific genetic variants that were apparently evolutionarily selected in response to specific dietary factors in the environment include lactose tolerance. Lactase persistence is one of the clearest examples of such a trait. Lactase persistence in adult life occurs in certain African populations where cattle husbandry occurred very early. Lactase persistence is also common in certain European populations (Fan *et al.*, 2016). A number of different genetic variants in the vicinity of the lactase gene have been associated with lactase persistence.

Occurrence of certain specific parasites in particular environments have also proved to be powerful selection forces. The best known of these are malaria parasites. It has long been known that certain hemoglobin variants, e.g. sickle cell hemoglobin mutation, and variants in certain enzymes including glucose-6-phosphate dehydrogenase (G6PD) are apparently specifically selected in regions with high incidence of malaria. The heterozygotes for the globin mutations and for the enzyme mutations are relatively more resistant to infection. However, homozygotes for these mutations and hemizygous males for the X-linked G6PD mutations suffer pathological effects of the variants.

Specific gene variants that impact skin color have also been shown to be under selective pressure, particularly in populations living in countries with little sun exposure, e.g. in northern Europe. These variants occur in genes involved in the synthesis and transport of melanin pigment: OCA2, TYR, TYRP1, SLC24A5 and SLC45A2.

Fan *et al.* (2016) emphasized particular genetic variants that were fixed in specific populations because of their selective advantage in prior eras, but may no longer be advantageous. One example they describe is a specific missense variant in a gene CREBF. This variant decreases energy usage and promotes energy storage and is likely to be advantageous during periods of short food supply. However, under conditions when food supplies are plentiful, the variant promotes fat storage and obesity. This particular variant occurs with high frequency in the Samoan population, who currently have the highest incidence of obesity in the world.

Another example of selective genomic influences connected with diet involves the AMY1 (amylase 1) gene that encodes an enzyme involved in starch digestion. Increased copy numbers of AMY1 have been observed in populations where the starch content of the diet is high, e.g. in Japan (Perry *et al.*, 2007).

Specific gene–environment interactions have been identified in cancer risk. Yang *et al.* (2010) reported that the genotypes of the ADH1B and ALDH2 genes (that encode enzymes involved in alcohol metabolism) affected the risk of esophageal cancer in Chinese and Japanese populations and that this risk was modified by alcohol consumption.

The Move Toward Personalized Precision Medicine

In establishing the Precision Medicine program at the National Institutes of Health (NIH) in the USA, the NIH leadership announced: "Far too many diseases have no proven means of prevention or effective treatments. We must gain better insights in to the biological, environmental and behavioral influences on diseases". Precision medicine projects will therefore be designed to take into account variability in genes, environment and lifestyle (Collins and Varmus, 2015).

40 Psychiatry

My interest in Human Genetics was initially stimulated during psychiatry rotation as a medical student and I have retained this interest throughout my career. I continue to be inspired by the modern emphasis on psychiatric disorders as brain disorders that are also impacted by environmental and social conditions.

New Insights through Comprehensive Genetic Studies

Extensive genomic and genetic studies have been carried out on large cohorts of patients diagnosed with neuropsychiatric disorders, on their family members and on control populations. A number of these studies have involved international teams of investigators, examples include studies by the Cross-Disorder Group of the Psychiatric Genetics Consortium (C-D Group, 2013; Ruderfer *et al*, 2014; Maier *et al*, 2015). Comprehensive genetic and genomic studies, coupled with family studies, have also been carried in Sweden. Examples of the latter were the Sandin *et al.* autism study (2014) that examined data from a Swedish population cohort of 2,049,973 children born between 1982 and 2006, and the study published in 2016 by Genovese *et al.*, in which data from 4,877 schizophrenia patients was published.

These studies have led to new insights into the inheritance and genetic mechanisms involved in psychiatric disorders; in addition they have provided information indicating that the fixed diagnostic categories in psychiatric disorders need to be revised.

Detailed studies reveal that within a specific family, different family members may be given different psychiatric diagnoses. Furthermore, a particular patient often has clinical features of more than one diagnosis (O'Donovan and Owen 2016).

Demonstration of Polygenic Risk in Psychiatric Disorders

The most robust insights that have emerged from comprehensive patient and family studies and genetic studies are that genetic risk in psychiatric disease is polygenic and that even in a specific individual, variants in a number of different genes impact disease risk. In addition, these studies have demonstrated that a range of different types of variants impact risk. These include genomic segmental variants (copy number variants), nucleotide sequence variants including common variants, rare variants, inherited variants and variants that arise *de novo* in patients.

The fact that damaging genetic variants occur with greater frequency in patients than in controls implies that underlying biological factors are involved in disorder causation. Detailed studies of genetic variants on the expression and function of genes have revealed that the larger category of genes that impact risk for psychiatric disease are genes that function at the neuronal synapses.

In a comprehensive study of autism associated damaging DNA variants and their functional impact, Krishnan *et al.* (2016) determined that the most abundant category of risk genes involved genes that encode products involved in synaptic transmission, neuronal plasticity, signaling processes and genes that play roles in brain development.

Genovese *et al.* (2016) carried out analysis of the function of gene products encoded by genes significantly impacted by rare damaging nucleotide variants in cases of schizophrenia. They determined that the majority of genes impacted functioned exclusively in the brain. However, some of the genes implicated functioned in more than one tissue. Most of the genes products altered by risk-inducing variants encoded synaptic functions.

They proposed that in future research, more complete analysis of proteins active within synaptic structures should be undertaken.

Genovese *et al.* emphasized that although their study concentrated on rare damaging variants, common variants also play roles in schizophrenia.

With respect to the implications of genetic studies for future development of more effective therapies for psychiatric diseases, Hyman (2016) emphasized the importance of understanding the underlying mechanisms affected by damaging genetic variants.

41 Aging

In an outstanding review of aging in 2013, Lopez-Otin *et al.* documented factors that play roles in aging and noted biological hallmarks of aging. These included genomic instability, telomere loss, epigenetic alterations, loss of proteostasis, deregulated nutrient sensing, mitochondrial dysfunction, cellular senescence, stem cell exhaustion and impaired intercellular communication.

Genomic Instability

Aging alterations occur at different levels in the genome. Based on studies of chromosomes in human female blood cells, a number of different investigators have reported loss of the human X chromosome associated with aging. Russell *et al.* (2007) reported that in females younger than 16 years of age, the X chromosome was absent from approximately 0.07% of cells. However, the frequency of X chromosome loss in cells from females older than 65 years was 7.3%.

It would be interesting to determine whether the X chromosome that remains after loss is the active X chromosome and whether the inactivated X chromosome was lost.

In an analysis of genomic segmental copy number variant (CNV) changes in aging and mortality, Kuningas *et al.* (2011) studied 6,892 individuals. They reported that a high burden of common CNVs larger than 500 kb in size was associated with a 4% higher mortality risk. These investigators identified two specific chromosome regions where deletions were associated with increased mortality risk. These regions included chromosome 11p15.5 and chromosome 14.21.3. They noted that 41 different genes map to chromosome 11p15.5, while no specific coding genes had been mapped to chromosome 14q21.3.

Lopez-Otin *et al.* reported that genomic defects in aging arise, in some instances, due to impairments in scaffolding elements, such as lamins that tether chromosomes to the nuclear membrane. Genetic defects in Lamin A predispose to the premature aging disorder Hutchinson–Gifford Progeria syndrome.

DNA damage occurs as a result of exogenous and endogenous factors that lead to DNA mutation. Damage also occurs through DNA breakage and through insertions into DNA of sequences from viruses and through movements of repetitive elements (transposons). A number of different DNA damage repair systems occur in humans; however, these systems may be overwhelmed if mutation is extensive. Genetic defects in specific DNA repair systems lead to premature aging associated with Werner syndrome.

Loss of telomeres at the ends of chromosomes (telomere attrition) occur during aging. There is evidence that after multiple cell divisions many cells can no longer restore telomeres at their ends, due to the absence of the enzyme telomerase. Telomerase is highly expressed in fetal cells and in adult germ cells. The enzyme telomerase is also expressed in tumor cells and this promotes their continued proliferation.

Epigenetic Changes in Aging

Epigenetic factors are factors that modify DNA without modifying the DNA code. These factors play key roles in modulating the expression of genes. Key epigenetic modifications include addition or removal of methyl groups to cytosine in DNA. Key epigenetic modifications of histones in DNA involve addition or removal of methyl groups and acetyl groups from histone tails.

Marioni *et al.* (2015) carried out studies to define the role of methylation in aging and mortality risk. Blood samples used were derived from three different cohorts, including 5,124 samples from the Framingham population cohort, 675 individuals from the US Veterans Normative Study and 614 individuals from an Australian population cohort. Ages of subjects in the different cohorts ranged between 66.3 years and 79.1 years. In order to measure DNA methylation, they extracted DNA from blood cells treated with bisulfite. Bisulfite converts cytosine residues in DNA to uracil, but leaves 5-methylcytosine residues unaffected. Uracil residues and

5-methylcytosine residues can be individually assessed through methylation microarray studies. The specific microarrays used in the Marioni *et al.* study assessed between 353 and 456 sites. Quantitative assessment of DNA was then carried out to develop a numerical methylation age. The methylation age minus the chronological age was then determined to develop a specific statistic. Based on results of their studies, Marioni *et al.* reported that differences between methylation age and chronological age were significant predictors of mortality risk. A difference between methylation age and chronological age of 5 years or greater was associated with a 16% increase in mortality risk.

Proteostasis

Proteostasis (protein homeostasis) involves processes that sense disturbances in solubility of proteins or their function and facilitates correction of these disturbances. Additional proteostasis mechanisms detect presence of protein aggregates and attempt to remove these (Kaushik and Cuervo, 2015).

The initial process, designed to attempt to refold unfolded non-functional proteins into correctly folded functional forms, involves the action of chaperones. These chaperones include small proteins known as heat shock proteins. Poor cellular energetics negatively impact chaperone activity, since that activity requires ATP as a source of energy. Kaushik and Cuervo also reported that specific modifications of proteins, such as excess glycosylation (addition of carbohydrate residues) impairs chaperone binding to unfolded proteins.

If proteins cannot be correctly folded, they enter into pathways designed to remove them. One such pathway is the ubiquitin–proteasomal pathway. Unfolded proteins are tagged with a small molecule (ubiquitin) and they are then transported to a specific cellular organelle, the proteasome, where they are degraded into their constituent amino acids.

Another process that degrades damaged proteins and damaged cellular organelles is autophagy. Autophagy is also required to rid cells of protein aggregates. Autophagy involves engulfment of damaged proteins and damaged cellular material and organelles into intracellular membranous structures, the endosomes. Subsequently, the endosomes with engulfed material fuse with lysosomes in the cell. Within the lysosomes, there are enzymes that ingest the engulfed substances. Failure to get rid of damaged proteins, protein aggregates and damaged cellular structures leads to age-related diseases including neurodegenerative diseases. Many age-related diseases are associated with accumulation of proteins with abnormal conformations.

Proteins with abnormal conformations can also accumulate in the endoplasmic reticulum prior to their release into the cytoplasm of the cells and these accumulated proteins can lead to endoplasmic reticulum stress and damage.

Mitochondrial Function Deterioration and Aging

There is evidence that mitochondrial dysfunction plays a major role in aging. This deterioration includes production of excessive quantities of reactive oxygen species and inadequate supplies of energy and ATP. Functional deterioration likely results from mitochondrial DNA mutations, impaired mitochondrial fission and fusion. Aging is associated not only with decreased mitochondrial bioenergetics but also with decreased generation of new mitochondria. Lane *et al.* (2015) noted that the health benefits of caloric restriction likely result in part from improved mitochondrial function.

Nutrient Sensing

There is evidence that nutrient sensing mechanisms are impaired in aging. Glucose level sensing through the insulin–insulin growth factor pathway plays a key role in maintaining metabolic balance. Other key pathways involved in maintenance of metabolic balance include the MTOR pathway, the adenosine monophosphate kinase (AMPK) pathway, and the Sirtuin pathway that senses levels of nicotinamide adenine dinucleotide (NAD). Deregulation of all of those pathways occurs in aging and dietary restriction promotes longevity through appropriate regulation of those pathways.

Cellular Senescence

Lopez-Otin *et al.* noted that cellular senescence is characterized by arrest of the cell cycle, so that cells no longer undergo cell division. Cell cycle arrest serves to impair division and proliferation of damaged cells. Senescence may also arise due to altered gene expression. Increased expression of the INK/ARF gene (p16) has been identified as a key factor that impairs cell division during aging.

Stem Cell Exhaustion

Impaired regeneration of stem cells in the bone marrow during aging leads to anemia and impaired immunological functions. Impaired generation of stem cells in the gastrointestinal tract also plays roles in defective gastro-intestinal function.

There is evidence that factors present in the blood of young animals can promote stem cell regeneration in various tissues, including the hip-pocampus of the brain. In addition, there is evidence that specific substances that accumulate in the blood during aging can damage stem cells.

Intercellular Communication

Lopez-Otin noted that intercellular communication is impaired in aging. A number of different factors play roles in intercellular communication. These include endocrine, neuro-endocrine, neuronal, metabolic factors and immunologic factors. Aberrant inflammatory responses occur in aging. It is not yet clear to what extent differences in the gut microbiome influence inflammatory responses in aging.

Brain Plasticity

The term brain plasticity is frequently used to refer to the changes in brain structure and function that occur in response to experience and learning. Initial studies were carried out in rats and mice exposed to diverse envi-ronmental inputs, including exercise and learning opportunities. Voss *et al.* (2013) reported that physical training and stimulating environments led to increases in generation and integration of new neurons and to increased blood flow to the brain.

Studies in humans, including older humans, have also been carried out by a number of different investigators. Hertzog *et al.* (2008) concluded: "The available evidence favors the hypothesis that maintaining an intellectually engaged and physically active lifestyle promotes successful aging". They also noted evidence that stress and psychological distress have negative effects on cognition.

Cognitive neuroscientists have illustrated another important aspect of brain plasticity in older adults. This involves the recruitment of alternate brain regions to perform specific tasks. Gutchess (2014) noted that plasticity "represents the potential for flexible recruitment of the brain, reflecting structural and functional changes sometimes as responses to learning and experience".

Stern (2009) and Kremen et al. (2012) emphasized that education, occupation, leisure activities and high quality social interactions have protective effects against age-related cognitive impairment. Jackson et al. (2011) reported that higher levels of conscientiousness had protective effects, while neuroticism was associated with an increased tendency to brain aging.

Neurogenesis in the Adult Brain

In their review of the generation of new neurons (neurogenesis) in the adult human brain, Kempermann et al. (2015) emphasized that this occurs in the dentate gyrus, a region of the hippocampus. Stem cells in the dentate gyrus generate granule cells. The precursor stem cells in the dentate gyrus have end-feet that make contact with endothelial cells of small blood vessels. These end-feet facilitate exchange of humoral factors from the small vessels to the precursor cells.

Kempermann et al. described three phases in the generation of new neurons. The first phase involves increased proliferation of stem cells in the dentate gyrus. The second phase is referred to as the post-mitotic maturation phase. This phase involves establishment of functional connections from the maturing dentate cells. These include growth of dendrites and axons and formation of synapses. The third phase involves maturation of dendritic spines and fine-tuning of function.

Mature granule cells in the dentate gyrus receive input from the entorhinal cortex and they send signals to the pyramidal cells located in a specific region of the hippocampus, the CA3 region. The entorhinal cortex is located in the temporal region of the brain. It is connected to the neocortex and to the hippocampus system. The entorhinal cortex–hippocampus system plays important roles in memory formation and consolidation. This system is also important in processing spatial orientation.

Kempermann *et al.* emphasized that adult hippocampal neurogenesis is of particular interest, since it adds functionality to the hippocampus known to be involved in cognitive functions and spatial navigation.

Costa *et al.* (2015) reported that there is abundant pre-clinical evidence that hippocampal neurogenesis is modulated by physiological stimuli, including physical and cognitive activity and emotional state.

Bouchard and Villeda (2015) drew attention to extensive evidence that factors including exercise, caloric restriction and changes in blood composition can counteract cognitive loss during aging. Studies on mice involving a technique termed parabiosis first illustrated the effects of humoral factors relative to aging.

Parabiosis involved generating vascular linkages between old and young mice and manipulation of the direction of blood flow. Investigators demonstrated that factors that circulated in the young mice could specifically counteract specific aging manifestations in older mice. Similarly, factors present in the blood of older mice could negatively impact functioning of young mice.

Further steps in these studies involved analysis of the specific factors present in the blood of young mice that counteracted aging effects.

McPherron *et al.* (2009) first reported that a specific growth factor, growth differentiation factor 11 (GDF11), derived from young animals reversed age-related impaired skeletal muscle and cardiac function in older animals. Katsimpardi *et al.* (2014) reported that administration of recombinant GDF11 to older mice had similar effects to those of young mouse blood on neurogenesis and vascular remodeling.

Smith *et al.* (2015) recently reported that levels of the protein beta-2-microglobulin were elevated in the circulation of older humans and older mice. Beta-2-microglobulin is a protein that is usually complexed with proteins of the HLA loci. Smith *et al.* also determined that exogenous beta-2-microglobulin impaired hippocampal neurogenesis and cognitive function in young mice.

Aging, Neurodegenerative Disease and Advances

Key concerns relative to aging, of course, center on the increased liability to neurodegenerative diseases as the years pass. Many of the most troubling neurodegenerative diseases are associated with increased precipitation and aggregation of specific proteins. These include beta amyloid in Alzheimer's disease, synuclein in Parkinson's disease and tau, that accumulates in those disorders and in other neurodegenerative diseases.

  Detailed studies on the solubility of these proteins and their precipitation relative to the protein concentration were carried out by Ciryam *et al.* (2013). In addition, platforms are being developed to readily test the efficacy of specific small molecules as inhibitors of aggregation (Saunders *et al.*, 2016). Clinical trials are also in progress to examine the value of molecules with antibody-like properties in clearing amyloid aggregates (Sevigny *et al.*, 2016).

42 Neurodegenerative Diseases

A number of different age-related neurodegenerative diseases, including Alzheimer's disease, Parkinson's disease, amyotrophic lateral sclerosis (ALS, Lou Gehrig's disease) and frontotemporal dementia, have certain histopathological and biological features in common. These include the accumulation of protein aggregates, protein misfolding and perturbations in the processes by which misfolded proteins are eliminated. In addition, there is evidence of impaired trafficking between cellular organelles and disturbed organelle function. Particularly important are defects in functioning of endosomes and lysosomes that are involved in taking up damaged proteins, and the structure and impaired function of mitochondria (Tofaris and Schapira, 2015). Together these impairments lead to degeneration of neurons. Another feature common to different neurodegenerative diseases is the accumulation of abnormal forms of the tau protein.

An important pathological feature common to these disorders is the occurrence of neuroinflammatory changes leading to alterations, and reactions that involve the glial cells in the brain (astrocytes and microglia). An important insight into the role of neuroinflammatory processes in neurodegenerative diseases was derived from the observation that heterozygous mutations in the TREM2 gene (that is only expressed in microglia in the brain) lead to neurodegenerative disease that can be associated with dementia. Homozygous mutations in this gene lead to a neuroinflammatory brain disease, with additional evidence of immune dysfunction, Nasu–Hakola disease (Ransohoff, 2016).

In addition to the common pathobiological features of neurodegenerative disease, there are also features that are specific to each specific neurodegenerative disease. Specific features can include the specific cell types involved, e.g. dopamine positive neurons are involved in Parkinson's disease. In ALS, motor neurons are specifically involved. The nature of the protein within aggregated structures tend also to be specific to a particular disease, thus beta amyloid containing plaques are specific to Alzheimer's disease and Lewy bodies that contain synuclein are specific to Parkinson's disease.

Evidence for Origin of Aggregates in One Region and Spread to Other Regions

Availability of neuroimaging with aggregate protein-specific markers has revealed that aggregate deposit often occurs initially in one part of the brain and that it slowly, progressively spreads to involve additional regions. There is also evidence for transneural spread of misfolded proteins. Braak and Del Tredici (2016) emphasized evidence for transneural spread of misfolded tau and alpha synuclein in Parkinson's disease.

In Alzheimer's disease, there is evidence that neurofibrillary tangles first appear in the hippocampus and then spread to other regions (Holtzman et al., 2016).

Clinical Features

Most of the neurodegenerative diseases apparently have long prodromal phases, during which time neurons degenerate but their loss is being compensated for within the brain. Braak et al. (2004) noted that typical manifestations of Parkinson's disease only occur after loss of 50% of dopaminergic neurons.

It is also important to note that familial cases of a specific neurodegenerative disease, for example Alzheimer's, and sporadic cases of that disease display many of the same manifestations. In general, clinical manifestations of the familial form of a specific neurodegenerative occur earlier in the life span, while in sporadic forms of that disease, the manifestations present later.

Family Studies and Genetics

Family studies and genetic studies have revealed that for each of the age related neurodegenerative diseases, there are familial forms due to monogenic gene defects and there are sporadic forms where no definitive evidence of Mendelian genetic inheritance is present.

Genome-wide association studies have revealed that the sporadic forms of neurodegenerative diseases are polygenic in origin. In each individual with a sporadic neurodegenerative disease, mutations in a number of different genes lead to the disorder and environmental factors also play roles. Genetic variants that lead to polygenic disease are frequently variants with relatively low damaging capacity and variants that are relatively common in the population. Disease results from the additive effects of the low risk variants.

In each of the different neurodegenerative disorders, distinct genes have been shown to carry variants. It will be useful therefore to consider each disease separately.

Alzheimer's Disease

The mutations that led to the familial monogenic forms of Alzheimer's disease most commonly involve genes that encode products involved in the processing of amyloid precursor proteins (e.g. presenilin enzymes), and lead to accumulation of the beta amyloid fragments derived from amyloid precursor proteins (De Strooper et al., 1998).

Mutations in at least 23 different genes have been found to be associated with sporadic late onset polygenic Alzheimer's disease. A number of studies have revealed that the most significant risk mutation occurs at the APOE gene locus, and the risk allele is APOE4. Other risk genes with variants that are encountered in a significant number of individuals include PICALM (that plays a role in uptake of lipoprotein in cells), CLU (a chaperone that transfers molecules between organelles in cells) and CRI, a cell receptor encoding gene (Lambert et al., 2013).

Extensive research has been carried out on the protein produced by the APOE locus. APOE is a lipoprotein carrying protein produced by many cells in the body, particularly by liver cells. In the brain, APOE is produced primarily by astrocytes and glial cells, however it is also produced by neuronal cells that are under stress (Mahley, 2016). There are three different allelic variants at the APOE locus: APOE2, APOE3 and APOE4. The three variant APOE proteins differ in their three dimensional structure due to amino acid residue differences between the three forms. Mahley (2016) reported that in neuronal cells APOE4 undergoes specific proteolytic breakdown, and this breakdown leads to the generation of a neurotoxic form of the protein that impairs mitochondrial function and also leads to abnormal phosphorylation of the protein tau.

Tambini et al. (2016) reported that the APOE4 variant protein impairs the normal interactions that take place between the endoplasmic reticulum and mitochondria.

There are active efforts underway to produce and analyze small molecule therapeutic agents to modify the amino acid interactions that lead to the abnormal APOE4 structure.

Parkinson's Disease

A number of genes have been shown to harbor mutations that lead to monogenic familial forms of Parkinson's disease. Mutations in the synuclein gene SNCA and the kinase gene LRRK2 play roles in autosomal dominant forms of Parkinson's disease. The genes PARKIN (involved in degradation of damaged proteins), PINK (important in mitochondrial function) and VPS35 (that is involved in endosomal function) play roles in autosomal recessive Parkinson's disease (Gasser, 2015).

There is evidence that sporadic Parkinson's disease is a polygenic disease, and that in each affected individual a number of medium risk or low risk variants have additive effects that lead to disease. Some of these low risk variants are different mutations in synuclein or in LRRK2. There are also low risk variants in 20 other genes that play roles, including variants in the glucocerebrosidase gene that impacts lysosomal function and variants in the MAPT gene that encodes the tau protein.

Amyotrophic Lateral Sclerosis (ALS)

ALS is characterized by dysfunction of upper motor neurons in the cerebral cortex and lower motor neurons of the brain stem and spinal cord. It has become clear that sporadic ALS is a polygenic disorder, implying that in each case deleterious variants in a number of different genes contribute to pathology. A number of the genes involved in ALS also play roles in other neurodegenerative diseases, including frontotemporal dementia and inclusion body myositis. A very important risk locus that undergoes alterations in familial and sporadic cases of ALS and in cases of frontotemporal dementia is a locus on chromosome 9, C9ORF72. The precise protein product of this locus has not been identified (Sabatelli *et al.*, 2016). Other risk genes involved in ALS include genes encoding proteins that play roles in mitochondrial function (SOD1, superoxide dismutase), CHCHD10, RNA binding proteins TARDP and FUS, VCP (an endoplasmic reticulum protein), and proteins involved in autophagy (digestion of degraded material). Other protein aggregates that occur in frontotemporal dementia include the ubiquitin-like proteins UBQLN2 and SQSTN.

Abnormal phosphorylation of tau protein also occurs in ALS, and particularly in frontotemporal dementia.

Tau Protein in Neurodegenerative Diseases

Accumulation of tau protein in the form of fibrillary deposits occurs in neurons and glial cells in a number of different neurodegenerative diseases. In addition, the form of tau that accumulates is often abnormally phosphorylated. Tau accumulates in Parkinson's disease and in diseases referred to as tauopathies; these include Pick's disease, corticobasil degeneration and supranuclear palsy. More than 50 different tau mutations have been identified in neurodegenerative diseases (Holtzman *et al.*, 2016).

Abnormal tau deposition also occurs secondary to brain infections (encephalopathies) or brain injury. In Alzheimer's disease there is apparently an interplay between amyloid beta deposition as plaques and tau precipitation in neurofibrillary tangles (Arendt, 2016).

Tau, encoded by the MAPT gene locus on chromosome 17, is present in many cells and is associated with microtubules and the actin cytoskeleton of cells. In neurons, there is evidence that tau plays a role in the movement of neurotransmitter receptors and in their endocytosis.

Holtzman *et al.* (2016) emphasized that tau pathology is the key driver of progression in Alzheimer's disease and in other neurodegenerative diseases. They noted that only in the 1980s were neurofibrillary tangles found to be composed of hyperphosphorylated insoluble proteins encoded by the MAPT locus.

Formation and aggregation of fibrillary tau is facilitated by the presence of other protein aggregates.

In neurodegenerative diseases described as tauopathies (Pick's disease, corticobasal disease (CBD) and primary supranuclear palsy, PSP), the primary aggregates present are aberrant tau proteins.

The MAPT gene maps to a segment on chromosome 17 that is liable to undergo inversion, leading to alteration of the exact order of marker loci in that region. This inversion give rise to two different haplotypes, H1 and H2, with different orders of markers. Neurodegenerative diseases with aberrant tau tend to occur more frequently in individuals with the H1 haplotype than in individuals with the H2 haplotype (Pittman et al., 2005). The MAPT locus gives rise on transcription to six different transcripts and protein isoforms.

Therapeutic Approaches

Holtzman et al. (2016) reported that therapeutic approaches to deal with tau pathologies include the use of inhibitors to promote degeneration of toxic forms of tau, and use of substances that attach carbohydrate residues to tau to prevent fibril formation. Tau is known to undergo other forms of modification that promote fibril formation and aggregation, one of these modification is acetylation. A specific small molecule, salsalate, inhibits this acetylation and is being considered for trials. Other approaches to therapy include the use of oligonucleotides to counteract mutations in MAPT that increase rates of precipitation. Immunotherapeutic approaches are also being considered to promote clearance of tau from neurons and its uptake by microglia.

Holtzman et al. emphasized the importance of ongoing in vivo imaging agents and biomarkers to monitor progression or improvement. Specific neuroimaging reagents are now available to detect amyloid beta precipitates and tau precipitates in the brain.

References

Arendt T, Stieler JT, Holzer M. (2016). Tau and tauopathies. Brain Res Bull 126(Pt 3): 238–292. doi: 10.1016/j.brainresbull.2016.08.018. PMID: 27615390.

Bainbridge MN, Wiszniewski W, Murdock DR, et al. (2011). Whole-genome sequencing for optimized patient management. Sci Transl Med 3(87):87re3. doi: 10.1126/scitranslmed.3002243. PMID:21677200.

Bouchard J, Villeda SA. (2015). Aging and brain rejuvenation as systemic events. J Neurochem 132(1):5–19. doi: 10.1111/jnc.12969. PMID:25327899.

Braak H, Ghebremedhin E, Rüb U, *et al.* (2004) Stages in the development of Parkinson's disease-related pathology. *Cell Tissue Res* **318(1):**121–34. PMID:15338272.

Braak H, Del Tredici K. (2016). Potential pathways of abnormal tau and α-synuclein dissemination in sporadic Alzheimer's and Parkinson's diseases. *Cold Spring Harb Perspect Biol* **8(11):** pii: a023630. doi: 10.1101/cshperspect.a023630. PMID:27580631.

Ciryam P, Tartaglia GG, Morimoto RI, *et al.* (2013). Widespread aggregation and neurodegenerative diseases are associated with supersaturated proteins. *Cell Rep* **5(3):**781–90. doi: 10.1016/j.celrep.2013.09.043. PMID 24183671.

Collins FS, Varmus H. (2015). A new initiative on precision medicine. *N Engl J Med* **372:**793–795. doi: 10.1056/NEJMp1500523.

Costa V, Lugert S, Jagasia R. (2015). Role of adult hippocampal neurogenesis in cognition in physiology and disease: pharmacological targets and biomarkers. *Handb Exp Pharmacol* **228:**99–155. doi: 10.1007/978-3-319-16522-6_4. PMID:25977081.

Cross-Disorder Group of the Psychiatric Genomics Consortium (2013). Identification of risk loci with shared effects on five major psychiatric disorders: a genome-wide analysis. *Lancet* **381(9875):**1371–9. doi: 10.1016/S0140-6736(12)62129-1. PMID:23453885.

De Strooper B, Saftig P, Craessaerts K, *et al.* (1998). Deficiency of presenilin-1 inhibits the normal cleavage of amyloid precursor protein. *Nature* **391(6665):** 387–90. PMID:9450754.

Fan S, Hansen EB, Lo Y, Tishkoff S. (2016). Going global by adapting local: A review of recent human adaptation. *Science* **354:** 54–58.

Gasser T. (2015). Usefulness of genetic testing in PD and PD trial: A balanced review. *J Parkinsons Dis* **5(2):**209–15. doi: 10.3233/JPD-140507. PMID:25624421.

Genovese G, Fromer M, Stahl EA, *et al.* (2016). Increased burden of ultra-rare protein-altering variants among 4,877 individuals with schizophrenia. *Nat Neurosci* **19(11):**1433–1441. doi: 10.1038/nn.4402. PMID:27694994.

Gutchess A. (2014). Plasticity of the aging brain: new directions in cognitive neuroscience. *Science* **346(6209):**579–82. doi: 10.1126/science.1254604. PMID:25359965.

Hall MA, Moore JH, Ritchie MD. (2016). Embracing complex associations in common traits: critical considerations for precision medicine. *Trends Genet* **32(8):**470–84. doi: 10.1016/j.tig.2016.06.001. PMID:27392675.

Hertzog C, Kramer AF, Wilson RS, Lindenberger U. (2008). Enrichment effects on adult cognitive development: can the functional capacity of older adults be preserved and enhanced? *Psychol Sci Public Interest* **9(1):**1–65. doi: 10.1111/j.1539-6053.2009.01034.x. PMID:26162004.

Hills E, Laverty CR. (1979). Electron microscope detection of papilloma virus particles in selected koilocytotic cells in a routine cervical smear. *Acta Cytol* **23(1)**:53–6. PMID:219647.

Hohne M, Schaefer S, Seifer M, *et al.* (1990). Malignant transformation of immortalized transgenic hepatocytes after transfection with hepatitis virus DNA. *EMBO J* **9**:1137–45. PMID:23233.

Holtzman DM, Carrillo MC, Hendrix JA, *et al.* (2016). Tau: From research to clinical development. *Alzheimers Dement* **12(10)**:1033–1039. doi: 10.1016/j.Jalz.2016.03.018. PMID:27154059.

Hyman SE. (2016). Back to basics: luring industry back into neuroscience. *Nat Neurosci* **19(11)**:1383–1384. doi: 10.1038/nn.4429. PMID:27786185.

Jackson J, Balota DA, Head D. (2009). Exploring the relationship between personality and regional brain volume in healthy aging. *Neurobiol Aging* **32(12)**:2162–71. doi: 10.1016/j.neurobiolaging.2009.12.009. PMID:20036035.

Karp CL, Wilson CB, Stuart LM. (2015). Tuberculosis vaccines: barriers and prospects on the quest for a transformative tool. *Immunol Rev* **264(1)**:363–81. doi: 10.1111/imr.12270.PMID:25703572.

Katsimpardi L, Litterman NK, Schein PA, *et al.* (2014). Vascular and neurogenic rejuvenation of the aging mouse brain by young systemic factors. *Science* **344(6184)**:630–4. doi: 10.1126/science.1251141. PMID:24797482.

Kaushik S, Cuervo AM. (2015). Proteostasis and aging. *Nat Med* **21(12)**:1406–15. doi: 10.1038/nm.4001. PMID 26646497.

Kempermann G, Song H, Gage FH. (2015). Neurogenesis in the adult hippocampus. *Cold Spring Harb Perspect Biol* **7(9)**:a018812. doi: 10.1101/cshperspect.a018812. PMID:26330519.

Klug A, Finch JT. (1968) Structure of viruses of the papilloma-polyoma type. IV Analysis of tilting experiments in the electron microscope. *J Mol Bio* **14**:31(1): 1–12. PMID: 4295242.

Kremen WS, Lachman ME, Pruessner JC, *et al.* (2012). Mechanisms of age-related cognitive change and targets for intervention: social interactions and stress. *J Gerontol A Biol Sci Med Sci* **67(7)**:760–5. doi: 10.1093/gerona/gls125. PMID 22570134.

Krishnan A, Zhang R, Yao V, *et al.* (2016). Genome-wide prediction and functional characterization of the genetic basis of autism spectrum disorder. *Nat Neurosci* **19(11)**:1454–1462. doi: 10.1038/nn.4353.

Kuningas M, Estrada K, Hsu YH, *et al.* (2011). Large common deletions associate with mortality at old age. *Hum Mol Genet* **20(21)**:4290–6. doi: 10.1093/hmg/ddr340. PMID:21835882.

Lambert JC, Ibrahim-Verbaas CA, Harold D, *et al.* (2013). Meta-analysis of 74,046 individuals identifies 11 new susceptibility loci for Alzheimer's disease. *Nat Genet* **45(12)**:1452–8. doi: 10.1038/ng.2802. PMID:24162737.

Lane RK, Hilsabeck T, Rea SL. (2015). The role of mitochondrial dysfunction in age-related diseases. *Biochim Biophys Acta* **1847(11):**1387–400. doi: 10.1016/j.bbabio.2015.05.021. PMID: 26050974.

López-Otín C, Blasco MA, Partridge L, et al. (2013). The hallmarks of aging. *Cell* **153(6):**1194–217. doi: 10.1016/j.cell.2013.05.039. PMID:23746838.

Maier R, Moser G, Chen GB, et al. (Cross-Disorder Working Group of the Psychiatric Genomics Consortium). (2015). Joint analysis of psychiatric disorders increases accuracy of risk prediction for schizophrenia, bipolar disorder, and major depressive disorder. *Am J Hum Genet* **96(2):**283–94. doi: 10.1016/j. ajhg.2014.12.006. PMID: 25640677.

Marioni RE, Shah S, McRae AF, Chen BH, et al. (2015). DNA methylation age of blood predicts all-cause mortality in later life. *Genome Biol* **16:**25. doi: 10.1186/s13059-015-0584-6. PMID:25633388.

Mahley RW. (2016). Apolipoprotein E: from cardiovascular disease to neurodegenerative disorders. *J Mol Med (Berl)* **94(7):**739–46. doi: 10.1007/s00109-016-1427-y. PMID:27277824.

McLaren MJ, Hawkins DM, Koornhof HJ, et al. (1975). Epidemiology of rheumatic heart disease in black schoolchildren of Soweto, Johannesburg. *Br Med J* **23;**3(5981):474–8. PMID: 1156827.

McPherron AC, Huynh TV, Lee SJ. (2009). Redundancy of myostatin and growth/ differentiation factor 11 function. *BMC Dev Biol* **9:**24. doi: 10.1186/1471-213X-9-24. PMID:19298661.

O'Donovan MC, Owen MJ. (2016). The implications of the shared genetics of psychiatric disorders. *Nat Med* **22(11):**1214–1219. doi: 10.1038/nm.4196. PMID:27783064.

Perry GH, Dominy NJ, Claw KG, et al. (2007). Diet and the evolution of human amylase gene copy number variation. *Nat Genet* **39(10):**1256–60. PMID:17828263.

Pittman AM, Myers AJ, Abou-Sleiman P, et al. (2005). Linkage disequilibrium fine mapping and haplotype association analysis of the tau gene in progressive supranuclear palsy and corticobasal degeneration. *J Med Genet* **42(11):** 837–46. PMID:15792962. doi:10.1136/jmg.2005.031377.

Ransohoff RM. (2016). How neuroinflammation contributes to neurodegeneration. *Science* **353(6301):**777–83. doi: 10.1126/science.aag2590. PMID:27540165.

Ruderfer DM, Fanous AH, Ripke S, et al. (Cross-Disorder Working Group of the Psychiatric Genomics Consortium). (2014). Polygenic dissection of diagnosis and clinical dimensions of bipolar disorder and schizophrenia. *Mol Psychiatry* **19(9):**1017–24. doi: 10.1038/mp.2013.138. PMID:24280982.

Russell LM, Strike P, Browne CE, Jacobs PA. (2007). X chromosome loss and ageing. *Cytogenet Genome Res* **116(3):**181–5. PMID: 17317957.

Sabatelli M, Marangi G, Conte A, *et al.* (2016). New ALS-related genes expand the spectrum paradigm of amyotrophic lateral sclerosis. *Brain Pathol* **26(2):**266–75. doi: 10.1111/bpa.12354. PMID:26780671.

Sandin S, Lichtenstein P, Kuja-Halkola R, *et al.* (2014). The familial risk of autism. *JAMA* **311(17):**1770–7. doi: 10.1001/jama.2014.4144. PMID:24794370.

Saunders JC, Young LM, Mahood RA, *et al.* (2016). An *in vivo* platform for identifying inhibitors of protein aggregation. *Nat Chem Biol* **12(2):**94–101. doi: 10.1038/nchembio.1988. PMID 26656088.

Sevigny J, Chiao P, Bussière T, *et al.* (2016). The antibody aducanumab reduces Aβ plaques in Alzheimer's disease. *Nature* **537(7618):**50–6. doi: 10.1038/nature19323. PMID:27582220.

Smith LK, He Y, Park JS, *et al.* (2015). β2-microglobulin is a systemic pro-aging factor that impairs cognitive function and neurogenesis. *Nat Med* **21(8):** 932–7. doi: 10.1038/nm.3898. PMID: 26147761.

Stern Y. (2009) Cognitive reserve. *Neuropsychologia* **47(10):**2015–28. doi: 10.1016/j.neuropsychologia.2009.03.004. PMID:19467352.

Sun S, Lu P, Gail MH, *et al.* (1999). Increased risk of hepatocellular carcinoma in male hepatitis surface antigen carriers with chronic hepatitis who have detectable urinary aflatoxin metabolite M1. *Hepatology* **30(2):** 379–383. PMID: 10421643

Tambini MD, Pera M, Kanter E, *et al.* (2016). ApoE4 upregulates the activity of mitochondria-associated ER membranes. *EMBO Rep* **17(1):**27–36. doi: 10.15252/embr.201540614. PMID:26564908.

Thomas L. (1974). *The Lives of the Cell, Notes of a Biology Watcher.* pp. 32–35. Re-published Penguin Books, 1996. ISBN-13:978-0140047431.

Tofaris GK, Schapira AH. (2015). Neurodegenerative diseases in the era of targeted therapeutics: how to handle a tangled issue. *Mol Cell Neurosci* **66(Pt A):**1–2. doi: 10.1016/j.mcn.2015.03.002. PMID:25749373.

Voss MW, Vivar C, Kramer AF, van Praag H. (2013). Bridging animal and human models of exercise-induced brain plasticity. *Trends Cogn Sci* **17(10):**525–44. doi: 10.1016/j.tics.2013.08.001. PMID:24029446.

Weiner J 3rd, Kaufman SH. (2014). Recent advances toward tuberculosis control: vaccines and biomarkers. *J Inter Med* **275(5):**467–480. doi: 10.1111/joim.12212 PMID:24635488

Yang SJ, Yokoyama A, Yokoyama T, *et al.* (2010). Relationship between genetic polymorphisms of ALDH2 and ADH1B and esophageal cancer risk: a meta-analysis. *World J Gastroenterol* **16(33):**4210–20. PMID:20806441.

Young BC, Levine RJ, Karumanchi SA. (2010). Pathogenesis of preeclampsia. *Annu Rev Pathol* **5:**173–92 doi.1146/annrev-pathol-12180n-102149 PMID:20078220.

PART VIII

The Future

43 Stem Cells and Pluripotent Stem Cells

In the future we can anticipate that pluripotent stem cells and differentiated cells derived from stem cells will increasingly be utilized to analyze the downstream effects of gene mutations and to develop and to test novel therapies.

The discovery by Takahashi and Yamanaka in 2006 that addition of four transcription factors could reprogram differentiated somatic cells to become pluripotent stem cells built on decades of prior work. In 2016, Takahashi and Yamanaka reviewed aspects of earlier work by developmental biologists that constituted the ground work for their discovery.

Somatic Cell Nuclear Fusion

In studies on frogs, John Gurdon (1962) revealed that when the nucleus from a differentiated somatic cell was transferred into an egg from which the nucleus had been removed, the resulting cell was pluripotent and could give rise to all the cell types of the embryo. Some cells derived from somatic cell nucleus transfer into enucleated eggs gave rise to tadpoles that eventually grew to adult frogs. This technique became known as somatic cell nuclear fusion (SCNT). It was clear that the enucleated egg contained factors that induced development of pluripotent cells from the transferred nucleus and that the resulting pluripotent cells could undergo cell division and subsequently give rise to differentiated cells.

In a 2009 commentary on nuclear reprogramming in somatic cell nuclear transfer, Gurdon reviewed mechanisms by which an enucleated egg or oocyte could reprogram a somatic nucleus. He noted that the oocyte accumulates reprogramming molecules, including Histone B4 and

Histone H1 subtypes. In addition, the oocyte accumulates molecules that can displace repressors from implanted nuclei.

Studies on Teratomas and Teratocarcinomas

Scientists and physicians have for many years been fascinated by teratomas and teratocarcinomas tumors that arise in gonads, testes or ovaries. These tumors contain a variety of different tissue types, including bone, skin, hair, muscle, etc.

Teratomas and teratocarcinomas also occur in mouse species. Kleinsmith and Pierce (1964) reported that a single cell from a teratoma or teratocarcinoma transplanted into the peritoneal cavity of the mouse could give rise to all of the tissues found in the original tumor from which the single cell was derived. This finding illustrated multipotentiality of the single cell.

In 1974 and in 1975, Martin and Evans reported that they had established cell line cultures from mouse teratocarcinoma cells. In 1981, Gail Martin reported that a single somatic cell from a mouse embryo could, when cultured in medium that was conditioned by growth of teratocarcinoma cell lines, give rise to pluripotent stem cells.

Embryonic Stem Cells Derived from the Blastocyst

Martin (1981), and Evans and Kaufman (1981) reported that they had established embryonic cell lines from mouse blastocysts. Thomson et al. (1998) reported that embryonic stem cell lines were established from human blastocysts.

The embryonic cells required special culture conditions and were grown on feeder layers of other types of cells.

Studies Leading up to the 2006 Discovery of Induced Pluripotency in Cells by Takahashi and Yamanaka

Takahashi and Yamanaka undertook studies to determine which genes were highly expressed in embryonic stem cells. They also analyzed factors used to promote maintenance of embryonic stem cells in culture. They narrowed down the list of important factors and then systematically determined the necessity of each of these factors to achieve pluripotency in embryonic cells. They eventually defined four factors that were essential to maintain pluripotency of embryonic cells. The four factors were transcription facts OCT3/4, KLF4, SOX2 and MYC, abbreviated OKSM. These four transcription factors were also found to convert human somatic cells into pluripotent stem cells. Delivery of the transcription factors into the cells was carried out by means of viral vectors.

In 2016, Takahashi and Yamanaka reported that in the first step in induction of pluripotency the OKSM transcription factors function as pioneer factors that bind to chromatin and lead to remodeling of chromatin regions.

The reprogramming efficiency was noted to be low and most of the OKSM treated cultures remained non-reprogrammed. However, reprogrammed cells could be purified from cultures based on the presence of specific antigens that were present on the reprogrammed cells; these included the SSEA1 antigen on reprogrammed mouse cells and the TRA1-60 antigen on reprogrammed human cells.

Vectors used to Transfer Pluripotency Factors

Retroviral vectors were initially used for reprogramming. More recently, vectors that do not become integrated into the chromosomes of the stem cells have been used. These vectors include the Sendai virus, that remains as an episome in the cells, separate from the chromosome.

There is now evidence that mRNA or proteins corresponding to transcription factors can be used to achieve pluripotency. Transcription factors other than OKSM have been used and pluripotency has also been achieved using small molecules.

Protocols to Establish Induced Pluripotent Stem Cells (IPS cells)

Hockemeyer and Jaenisch (2016) emphasized that the publication of extensive protocols for the induction of pluripotent stem cells from somatic cells and for the maintenance of pluripotent cells have facilitated progress in the field.

In addition, extensive studies have been carried out on the use of growth factors and cofactors that induce pluripotent cells to differentiate into particular cell types. One important factor to take into account, however, is that the application of specific differentiation factors leads to generation of only a low percentage of differentiated cells. It is important that specific markers of differentiated cells be identified. Such markers can then be used to identify appropriately differentiated cells from the other cells present in cultures.

Use of IPS Cells as Models to Study Disease-associated Cellular Defects

Skin biopsies from patients with monogenic diseases have been used to derive stem cells and differentiated cells to analyze the biochemical and biological effects of specific mutations on functions of tissue-specific cell types. The differentiated cells can then be used to study the downstream effects of specific mutations. Importantly, such cells can also be used to investigate the utility of particular therapeutic agents.

Hockemeyer and Jaenisch (2016) noted that IPS techniques have enabled progress in modeling of human neurodegenerative diseases. One example presented was a study on the neurodegenerative disease amyotrophic lateral sclerosis (ALS). One form of ALS is due to mutations in the SOD1 gene that encodes superoxide dismutase. IPS cells derived from patients with SOD1 mutations differentiated into neurons, revealing a previously unknown downstream effect of SOD1 mutations, namely a functional deficit in potassium channels that led to specific electrophysiological abnormalities and hyper-excitability of neurons. When the IPS-derived SOD1 neurons were treated with a specific medication that functions as a potassium channel agonist, the hyper-excitability defect was corrected.

Wainger et al. (2014) determined that mutations in certain other genes led to ALS, and that mutations in the C9ORF72 and FUS genes also led to the abnormal motor neuron physiology that responded to treatment with the same potassium channel agonist.

McNeish et al. (2015) emphasized that new IPS cell models for human diseases are regularly being reported. For several of these diseases, correction of physiological defects with specific treatments has also been reported.

Pluripotent Stem Cells and Cardiomyopathies

Ross *et al.* (2016) published studies on the use of IPS cell-derived cardiomyocytes to study the impact of specific mutations associated with cardiomyopathy. They determined that components in four specific signaling pathways are required for differentiation of cardiac myocytes. These pathways include the transforming growth factor beta, activin, nodal and fibroblast growth factors. Identification of differentiated cardiac myocytes can be accomplished through analysis of specific markers TNNT2 (cardiac troponin 2) and MEF2 (myocyte enhancer factor 2).

In addition to derivation of monolayers of differentiated myocytes, Ross *et al.* noted that it was also of value to generate and study embryoid bodies. Embryoid bodies are 3-dimensional aggregates of differentiated cells. Within embryoids, a heterogeneous population of differentiated cells sometimes develops and these structures can mimic organ-like structures.

Ross *et al.* reported that IPS cell-derived cardiac myocytes from patients with the cardiac myosin gene defect MHY7 arg442gly revealed disorganized sarcomeres and increased concentrations of intracellular calcium. MYH7 mutation leads to hypertrophic cardiomyopathy. IPS cell-derived cardiac myocytes from patients with mutations in cardiac troponin 2 TNNT2 arg72trp showed abnormal sarcomere alignment and abnormal actinin distribution. TNNT2 mutations are associated with dilated cardiomyopathy. Studies on IPS cell-derived cardiomyocytes are valuable in confirming the pathogenicity of specific nucleotide variants found on sequencing the DNA of patients with cardiomyopathy. Differentiated cardiomyocytes provide opportunities for testing of specific medications to improve cardiac function.

Funakoshi *et al.* (2016) emphasized that although IPS-derived cardiomyocytes can be developed, additional studies will be required before such cells could, for example, be used to repair hearts damaged by myocardial infarction. Key problems are apparently related to the integration of the derived cardiomyocytes into heart muscle tissue.

IPS Cells and Studies of the Aging Process

Lemey *et al.* (2015) reported that protocols have been developed to establish IPS cells from older individuals, including centenarians.

Lopez-Otin *et al.* (2013) defined cellular hallmarks of aging. These including epigenetic changes, alteration in gene expression, genomic instability, telomere loss and altered nutrient sensing. Lemey *et al.* reported that additional features of aging include loss of stem cells and decreased stem cell regenerative capacity. In senescent cells, cell cycle arrest is common. Hayflick (1961) described the phenomenon of progressively decreased rates of cell proliferation of aging cells in culture. Blackburn *et al.* (2006) attributed the loss of proliferative capacity of senescent cells to a decreased ability of these cells to form telomeres due to lack of telomerase, the ribonucleoprotein that forms telomeres at the end of chromosomes.

Other factors responsible for cellular senescence include increased production of reactive oxygen species and peroxides due to altered mitochondrial metabolism. Another feature of senescent cells is increased production of specific oncogene products, e.g. P16INK and p21CIP. One of the hallmarks of senescent cells is the presence of altered chromatin. These alterations are detected microscopically and are reported as senescence-associated heterochromatin foci, SAHF (Kuilman *et al.*, 2010).

Lapasset *et al.* (2011) succeeded in deriving induced pluripotent cells from senescent somatic cells through the use of six transcription factors, including OKSM and in addition Nanog and Lin28. The latter two factors were known to promote induction of pluripotency through experiments of Yu, Thomson *et al.* (2007).

Lemey *et al.* (2015) also used these six transcription factors to establish induced pluripotent stem cells from somatic cells of older individuals. They demonstrated that in the IPS cells, the P16INK and p21CIP oncogenes were down-regulated. Furthermore, in the reprogrammed cells, the mean length of telomeres increased and the senescence-associated heterochromatin foci disappeared. One important step will be to determine if these IPS cells can be differentiated into specific tissue type cells.

Pluripotent Stem Cells and Regenerative Medicine

Several very important assurances will be required before IPS cells can be used directly on patients. Clearly, cells need to be free of harmful viruses or contaminants. Trounson and De Witt (2016) emphasized that there needs to be clear evidence that when cells are transplanted *in vivo* they will be integrated into the tissue and will function correctly. Another important consideration is that cells will not elicit an abnormal immune response in the patients. Processes that lead to generations of tissue-specific cell types from the patient's own IPS cells are unlikely to lead to immune response. Another important consideration is that sufficient numbers of fully differentiated IPS cells must be available.

Trounson and DeWitt noted that the IPS cell treatment approaches that are most advanced in clinical trials include use of retinal pigment epithelium-like cells, that have entered phase II clinical trials for treatment of macular degeneration.

Essential evidence required prior to therapy initiation includes studies in animal models (usually rodent models) that the transplanted IPS cell type will integrate into damaged tissue and function correctly.

Cellular Therapies using Bone Marrow-derived Cells

Bone marrow cells used in therapies include hematopoietic stem cells and bone marrow mesenchymal cells. Bone marrow mesenchymal cells are derived from the sinusoidal blood vessels in bone marrow (Bianco *et al.*, 2013). These cells can be cultured from bone marrow as adherent cells and can differentiate into cartilage or bone. Clinical uses for these cells are being explored (Trounson and DeWitt).

Hematopoietic stem cells or bone marrow transplants are established therapies in certain forms of cancer.

An important development during the past 25 years has been the establishment of banks of umbilical cord blood stem cell banks. An additional advance in this area was reported by Wagner *et al.* (2016), who described methods to expand the numbers of umbilical cord blood cells in culture.

Tissue and Organ Chips

Advances in cell biology, in microfabrication and in microfluidic technologies have facilitated development of functional models of specific tissues and organs (Esch *et al.*, 2014). The models, sometimes referred to as organs on chips are of particular value in preclinical drug testing.

Esch *et al.* reported micro-engineered models have been built to recapitulate the structural and functional complexity of liver, lung, kidney, bone and other organs.

44 Gene Editing

This refers to the modification of specific genome sequence targets through the use of nucleases, enzymes that cut DNA. Gene editing can be used as a method to modify genes in *in vitro* conditions, to assess the functions of specific genes and to assess the downstream effects of specific gene mutations.

In clinical genetics, the main interest lies in the possibilities for using gene editing to remove mutant nucleotides to restore gene functions. Early proposed targets for gene editing include mutations that could be corrected in readily accessible cells, for example bone marrow stem cells.

Gene Editing Technologies

The key functional component in gene editing involve the nuclease enzymes that can cut DNA. An important factor for genome editing in vertebrates is that the gene editing system must achieve excision of double stranded DNA, at a particular target site. This cleavage will result in nucleotides at the cleavage site. The double stranded cleaved DNA will then undergo healing. Healing may be achieved by end joining, i.e. the cleaved ends will rejoin without the excised nucleotides. An alternate method of healing can be accomplished if extrinsic sequence is available that overlaps the two ends. Availability of such a DNA segment would permit healing by a process known as homologous recombination.

Earlier gene editing methodologies involved the use of Zinc finger nuclease (ZFNs) and TALENS, transcription activator-like effector nucleases. More recently, a more efficient form of gene editing has become available, this system is known as the CRISPR Cas9 system. The CRISPR Cas9 system uses RNA to target the cleavage site. Specific vectors have been designed to facilitate delivery of a guide RNA to a target site in the genome. The guide RNA containing CRISPR relates sequence crRNA and tracrRNA to provide the scaffold necessary for Cas9 nuclease binding. The guide RNA also contains a 20 nucleotide targeting sequence. In selecting the targeting sequence, it must lie 20 nucleotides upstream of a so-called PAM sequence. The PAM sequence NGG (any nucleotide followed by two guanine nucleobases) must be in the host genome. In the CRISPR Cas editing system, the guide sequence and the targeting sequence are RNA-based and the targeting is dependent on simple base pairing between the engineered RNA and the target DNA (Sander and Joung, 2014). Following this binding and positioning of the Cas9 nuclease cleavage, a double stranded DNA break will result. Crispr Cas editing can be designed to delete one or more nucleotides from DNA. The break in the DNA strand can be repaired by end joining of the cleaved fragments or by insertion of a sequence that matches the sequences on either side of the DNA cleavage.

Specificity of targeting is therefore very important. Sander and Joung reported that complementarity between the targeted DNA sequence and the guide RNA must be at least 17 nucleotides in length and often 20 nucleotides are selected. Specific programs of nucleotide sequences are available online to facilitate appropriate selection of target sites and to minimize off-target effects.

The editing system must be efficiently delivered to the nucleus of the cell to be edited. Plasmids are often used to carry the guide sequence with targeting RNA and Cas9 nuclease into the nucleus. However, electroporation techniques are sometimes used to avoid the use of plasmids, that are viral-like entities. In some studies, cell penetrating peptides that bind to the guide RNA have been used to facilitate delivery (Maeder and Gersbach, 2016).

Most gene editing experiments have been carried out *in vitro*, e.g. on cultured host cells or stem cells. In animal models, vectors with organ and tissue specific capacities have sometimes been used *in vivo* to deliver gene targeting systems.

The most direct gene editing experiments involve cleavage that results in knockout of a specific gene segment. This strategy was applied to human T cells to knockout the CCR5 co-receptor that binds the HIV virus.

In vitro experiments have been carried out to explore the feasibility of using gene editing to treat hemoglobinopathies, such as sickle cell anemia and thalassemia. Several investigators have used gene editing to treat hemoglobinopathies involving the beta globin locus, by enhanced expression of gamma globin. Gamma globins are expressed almost exclusively in late fetal life and expression ceases shortly after birth. Hematologists have observed that in certain patients with hemoglobinopathies due to mutations in the beta globin gene, e.g. sickle cell beta globin mutations or beta globin thalassemia, mutations also had alterations in the gamma gene promoter regions or in the sequences that control gamma expression; if these mutations led to persistence of gamma globin expression, then patients had much less severe effects of the beta globin mutations. The condition, characterized by lifelong continuation of gamma globin expression, is referred to as hereditary persistence of fetal hemoglobin (HPFH).

Researchers have used gene editing techniques to artificially induce HPFH. Traxler *et al.* (2016) used Crispr Cas editing to modify promoter sequences in the gamma globin genes so that gamma globin synthesis continued, even in adult cells.

An important regulatory gene sequence region that controls gamma globin shut-off after fetal life is a sequence that binds the transcription factor BCL11A. Ye *et al.* (2016) used CRISPR Cas technology to delete the BCL11A binding site in hematopoietic progenitor stem cells. Deletion of this binding site led the cells to increase production of gamma globin. They proposed that this strategy might provide an efficient approach to edit patient-derived cells, that can then be re-transplanted into the patient.

Editing methodologies have been designed to correct genomic changes that lead to disease. Hemophilia A is a condition associated with abnormal bleeding tendencies that occurs in 1 in 5,000 males in the USA. Hemophilia A is due to defects in the Factor VIII gene that is located on the X chromosomes. In approximately half of the affected cases of hemophilia, there is a structural genomic change characterized by inversion of the intron sequence in a specific position. This flip in sequence alters the linearity of the nucleotide sequence and impairs appropriate transcription and translation.

Park *et al.* (2015) used CRISPR Cas gene editing technique and patient-derived pluripotent cells to correct the inversion of the Factor VIII gene. They also demonstrated that endothelial cells could be differentiated from the corrected stem cells. In a mouse model of hemophilia A, administration of the corrected cells could correct the Factor VIII deficiency and correctly treat the disease.

Clinical Trials of Gene Edited Cells

The first clinical trial of CRISPR Cas9 edited cells to be approved in the USA was related to T lymphocyte modification to treat cancer. A trial to determine the safety of edited T cells in certain patients with cancer was approved in June 2016 (Reardon, 2016).

45 Antisense Oligonucleotides

It is likely that in the next years there will be progress in identifying specific nucleotide mutations that lead to particular genetic diseases. It is also likely that therapies will be designed to neutralize the effects of these mutations. Antisense oligonucleotides represent one form of therapy that will be applied.

Antisense oligonucleotides are short chains of oligonucleotides in single strands that can bind to short segments of mRNA and prevent that segment from being translated. In some cases, the binding of the antisense oligonucleotide to mRNA leads to destruction of that mRNA by a ribonuclease enzyme.

An antisense RNA was recently given FDA approval in the USA for treatment of Duchenne Muscular dystrophy due to a specific mutation in exon 51 of the dystrophin gene. This mutation leads to a premature termination, so that transcription and generation of mRNA cannot continue beyond this point. The dystrophin gene has 79 exons, so termination of transcription at exon 51 leads to a transcript that is missing 28 exons and is non-functional.

It turns out, however, that exon 51 is not essential for dystrophin function. Antisense oligonucleotides that block exon 51 allow the generation of a transcript that can be translated into a functional dystrophin protein.

One problem with antisense oligonucleotide therapies is that getting the antisense oligonucleotides into the appropriate cell type at high enough concentrations can be problematic. However, a form of antisense oligonucleotide in clinical trials for muscular dystrophy was found to reach therapeutic levels following intravenous injection: https://www.sciencedaily.com/releases/2016/09/160920095640.htm.

Antisense oligonucleotides have also been investigated to treat a number of other genetic diseases due to specific mutations, e.g. spinal muscular atrophy. The antisense oligonucleotide in clinical trial to treat this disorder is a splice switching antisense oligonucleotide. For treatments of spinal muscular atrophy, the splice switching antisense oligonucleotide does not target the mutation in the SMN1 gene. Instead, it targets a specific splice site that is normally present in the SMN2 gene, a highly similar gene A functional SMN2 gene product is usually not expressed in humans because a full length functional version of the SMN2 gene product cannot be produced. Administration of the splice switching oligonucleotide leads to SMN2 production and to significant improvement in the neurological manifestations in a mouse model of spinal muscular atrophy. The splice switching oligonucleotide Nusinersen is in clinical trials in the USA (Hache et al., 2016).

46 Towards the Future of Cancer Diagnosis and Therapy

Extensive studies are ongoing to analyze tumor DNA through next generation sequencing and to match mutations with specific therapies that target tumor-specific mutations. One such program is the USA National Cancer Institute (NCI) trial designated MATCH (Molecular analysis for therapy choice). This trial currently specifically enrolls patients with advanced solid tumors or lymphomas that are not responding to standard therapies. The goal is to search for genetic mutations that may respond to specific target therapies. In patients recruited to the MATCH trial, mutation testing and drug costs are covered by the NCI (https://www.cancer.gov/about-cancer/treatment/clinical-trials/nci-supported/nci-match).

As of May 2016, the MATCH program had 24 different target therapies available. Targeted cancer therapies are drugs or substances that block the growth and spread of cancer by interfering with specific molecular targets and altered processes that are present in tumor cells but not in normal cells. The targeted molecules and processes arise as a result of mutations in the tumors and are often drivers of tumor growth. One example of a process that can be successfully targeted therapeutically is the abnormally high expression of a particular receptor on tumor cells, e.g. the epidermal growth factor receptor HER2 in some forms of breast cancer.

Target mutations are sometimes referred to as actionable mutations or driver mutations. As research progresses more driver/actionable mutations will be identified and more drugs that target such mutations will be found. Additional appropriately tested drugs will be added to the MATCH therapies.

It is also important to note that genomic studies have sometimes revealed that tumors with identical histological features sometimes have different genomic alterations and that these may prompt different targeted therapies despite histological similarities.

Targeted Therapies in Clinical Use for Cancer

Specific therapies developed to target molecules that are mutated (and therefore facilitate the growth of tumor cells) include antibodies and specific chemicals designated as small molecules. Monoclonal antibodies used in cancer therapy have -mab at the end of the name. Small molecules are often inhibitors and they have -ib at the end of the name.

Liquid Biopsies: Analysis of Circulating Tumor Nucleic Acids

Important new developments that are particularly advantageous in assessing the response of tumors to therapies include the development of techniques to examine tumor derivatives in the circulation and in other body fluids.

A number of different tumor-derived components enter the circulation and certain body fluids; these include tumor cells, exosomes and nucleic acids from tumors. Most progress has been made in methods to isolate and analyze exosomes and tumor-derived nucleic acids (Hofman and Popper, 2016).

Exosomes

Exosomes are cell-derived vesicles that are enclosed in a lipid bilayer. Melo et al. (2015) reported that cancer cell-derived exosomes are particularly rich in a proteoglycan, glypican 1. The presence of this substance on exosomes facilitates their purification from blood and body fluids.

Exosomes are vesicles that form in cells and contain cellular molecules including proteins and nucleic acids (including genomic DNA fragments and RNA). Exosomes fuse with lysosomes in cells; in lysosomes the cell products are degraded. Exosomes also fuse with the membranes that surround cells and in that process, exosomes enter the extracellular spaces and subsequently enter the circulation or other body fluids.

Studies of DNA in exosomes can be carried out to search, for example, for mutations characteristic of a certain tumor. Cell-free DNA and DNA not contained in exosomes can also be isolated from circulating blood or body fluids, including urine or cerebrospinal fluid, and this can be used for sequencing.

Pan et al. (2015) utilized cerebrospinal fluid (CSF) to detect evidence of the presence of tumor-specific cell-free DNA in patients with primary or metastatic brain tumors. Wang et al. (2015) carried out studies in CSF to detect tumor-specific DNA. They emphasized the importance of CSF DNA studies for disease monitoring in cases with brain tumors.

Siravegna et al. (2015) reported that mutations leading to therapeutic resistance were readily detected in cell-free circulating DNA.

Studies of cell-free tumor DNA have revealed that early studies of circulating tumor products may be warranted, even for early diagnosis of cancer. Martin et al. (2016) reported that surgical interventions (including biopsy) are associated with increased concentrations of circulating tumor cells.

Cancer Metastases

Exosomes

There is evidence that proteins, RNA, DNA and other molecules contained within exosomes that are released from tumors may prime sites in distant tissues to facilitate subsequent colonization of these tissue tumor cells. Lyden and collaborators (see Hoshino et al., 2015) also proposed that integrin proteins contained in exosomes play important roles in preparing tissues for subsequent colonization by tumor cells.

Cheung and Ewald (2016) provided evidence that the development of tumor metastases was dependent on seeding of distant sites by clusters of tumor cells. They also noted that such clusters often contain tumor cells of different clonal composition.

Changes in Metabolism in Tumors

Studies by different investigators over many decades have demonstrated that metabolism is altered in tumors. In a 2016 review of metabolism in cancer, Sullivan et al. reported that in certain tumors, levels of specific metabolites may be altered. These metabolites include fumarate, succinate aspartate and reactive oxygen species. In addition, oncometabolites, unusual metabolites, may be found in certain tumors. The oncometabolite 2-hydroxyglutarate (D2HG) occurs in certain tumors as a result of mutations in the genes that encode the enzymes isocitrate dehydrogenase 1 or isocitrate dehydrogenase 2.

Therapeutic approaches to cancer treatment include blocking of oncometabolite production and suppressing the metabolic pathways on which cancer cells are particularly dependent.

Immunotherapy in Cancer

Careful decoding of basic immunology and searches for the relevance of different aspects of immunology to cancer have led to important breakthroughs in cancer treatment. One of the mechanisms by which tumors avoid immune suppression is to upregulate the expression of specific molecules that impair the function of killer T cells that invade the tumor.

Immune Modulators

In 1996, Leach, Krummel and Allison identified one specific molecule that is produced by tumors and that suppresses T cell function. This molecule was designated as Cytotoxic T-Lymphocyte Associated Protein 4 (CTLA4). They demonstrated that antibodies that blocked the function of CTLA4 led to disappearance of mouse tumors. Following extensive clinical trials, the USA FDA approved anti-CTLA4 antibody Ipilimumab for treatment of melanoma tumors.

Studies by several groups including Freeman et al. (2000) reported finding another molecule, PD1 (programmed death 1) produced by tumors that impaired lymphocyte functions. Subsequently, two additional molecules were identified that bind to PD1, these were designated PD1-L1 and PD1-L2.

Chen and Han (2015) reviewed the PD1/PDL pathway and the role of this pathway in inhibiting T cell response to antigens. Under normal circumstances, these molecules serve to suppress the organism's response to self-antigens. In fact, mice deficient in PDL1 develop autoimmune disease.

PD1 is expressed on many cell types and in normal tissue. PDL1, however, has more limited expression in normal tissues. However, PDL1 was found to be abundantly expressed by a number of different cancerous tumors. Blocking of PDL1 by antibodies was found to lead to tumor regression. In 2012, Topalian *et al.* reported on the safety and efficacy of anti-PD1L antibodies in cancer therapy.

The PD1/PDL pathway allows tumor cells to resist detection by the immune sytem. PD1 and PDL1 are referred to as immunomodulators. Several antibodies that specifically impact these immunomodulators have been approved for clinical use by the FDA.

In an August 2016 review, Dijkstra *et al.* noted that use of antibodies against CTLA4 and antibodies against PD1/PDL1 had achieved success in treating a number of different malignancies. However, not all patients treated with these antibodies responded. In addition, side effects to therapy sometimes occurred. Furthermore, costs of therapy were high. For the latter reasons, Dijkstra *et al.* emphasized that prior assessment of the likelihood of successful response to treatment with these antibodies should be assessed in prior studies. They note that therapeutic outcome is likely determined in part by the degree of "foreignness'" of the tumor, that is how many novel molecules that constitute antigens are produced as a result of mutations in the tumor. Genomic sequencing of tumors can facilitate assessment of the level of mutations in tumors. Another determinant of treatment success with immunomodulator antibodies has to do with the degree of lymphocyte invasions by the tumor.

There is also evidence that specific factors produced by macrophage cells (phagocytic cells) also modulate the immune response.

Adaptive Cell Transfer and Immunotherapy

Studies on melanoma tumors were among the first to reveal that tumors are often invaded by large numbers of lymphocytes with anti-tumor properties. Rosenberg and Restifo (2015) established procedures to isolate lymphocytes from tumors and to establish cultures of these lymphocytes *in vitro*. They reported that addition of the growth factor IL2 stimulated *in vitro* growth of the lymphocytes in tumor cultures. The lymphocytes with anti-tumor properties were primarily T cells of the CD8 positive and the CD4 positive type. Importantly, the tumor invading lymphocytes were found to recognize specific tumor antigens.

The observation that reinfusion of the cultures of tumor-derived lymphocytes could destroy melanoma tumors in some patients has led to the exploration of so-called adoptive cell therapy for cancer treatment.

Tumor Antigens

Specific mutations that occur within tumors can give rise to proteins with new amino acid sequences and to proteins that are not recognized as self by the immune system in that patient. Rosenberg and Restifo reported that degradation of these novel proteins to peptides may give rise to novel peptides that enter specific antigen presenting cells in the patients. If these novel peptides then associate with components of the major histocompatibility complex (MHC), the novel antigens can be presented on the surface of the antigen presenting cells. There they bind to specific receptors on T lymphocytes and elicit cytotoxic responses that destroy the tumor cells that produced the novel antigens.

Procedures to stimulate lymphocytes and the cytotoxic response include specific introduction of peptides from novel tumor antigens into patient's antigen presenting cells.

Engineered T Cell Receptors in Cancer Therapy

Specifically engineered T cell receptors have been developed in the laboratory. Fesnak *et al.* (2016) reported that engineered chimeric antigen receptors, CARs, do not require binding to MHC molecules to be presented on antigen presenting cells. This is important because tumors often downregulate the production of MHC components. CARs are composed of components derived from antibody producing B cells and a specific component of the T cell receptor.

A key factor in adaptive cell transfer is the recognition and isolation from the tumors of mutant proteins that are likely to have significant antigen activity.

Cancer Vaccines

Cancer vaccines are classified as prophylactic vaccines and therapeutic vaccines. Prophylactic vaccines have been developed against specific cancer causing viruses. A very important vaccine was development to counteract the Human Papilloma virus (HPV). This virus causes cervical cancer, genital cancer and nasopharyngeal cancer. Another important prophylactic cancer vaccine is the vaccine that prevents hepatitis B infection, that can lead to liver cancer.

Therapeutic cancer vaccines are designed to activate T immune cells that will destroy tumor cells or to stimulate the production of antibodies that will bind to tumor cells and promote their destruction.

Production of cancer vaccines requires the isolation of specific antigens from cancer cells. These antigens can include proteins and glycoproteins. RNA or DNA corresponding to genes that stimulate production of immunogenic products can also be used for vaccine production.

The USA National Cancer Institute reports that the first cancer vaccine approved for therapy was a vaccine to treat metastatic prostate cancer. In addition, there are active clinical trials in place for treatment of several other forms of cancer, including cancers of the bladder, brain, breasts, colon, lymphoid systems and lung.

Experiments are also ongoing in the use of whole cancer cells and dendritic cells to produce cancer vaccines. Dendritic cells are present in tissues that underlie body surfaces, including mucosa in the airways and gastrointestinal surfaces; in addition they are present in the circulation. Dendritic cells can phagocytose particles (including antigens) and in this process they are activated to form mature dendritic cells that then migrate to lymphoid tissues in various locations and in the spleen. In lymphoid tissues, mature dendritic cells that present antigens bound to histocompatibility molecules on their surface activate lymphocytes.

Lipid-complexed Nucleic Acids, Dendritic Cells and Cancer Immunotherapy

Kranz et al. (2016) reported a new approach to immunotherapy of tumors. This approach was based in part on the close proximity of antigen presenting dendritic cells to lymphocytes. They demonstrated further that molecules such as RNA, when complexed to specific lipid carrier molecules, can be injected and make their way to dendritic cells and lymphoid tissues. Furthermore, when RNA was complexed to lipid and to interferon and was ingested by dendritic cells, the interferon stimulated maturation of the dendritic cells. Any RNA that encodes an antigen can readily be synthesized. The lipid that is associated with RNA in the complexes serves to protect the

RNA from degradation by RNAse enzymes. In pre-clinical trials, Kranz et al. (2016) determined, through histological and immunostaining methods, that this new class of RNA vaccines they developed made their way to lymph nodes, spleen and bone marrow.

Kranz et al. reported successful treatment of advanced melanoma through use of RNA corresponding to tumor antigens and complexed with interferon and lipids. Following this treatment, all patients developed a T cell response against tumor antigens.

The Cancer Moonshot

An exciting program with significant implications for cancer therapy was established in the USA in January 2016. In response to presidential announcement of the program, a Blue Ribbon Panel was established to guide the direction of the program. The report of the ten key initiatives in this program was made available by the National Cancer Institute in September 2016 (https://www.cancer.gov/research/key-initiatives/moonshot-cancer-initiative/blue-ribbon-panel).

These initiatives are summarized below.

A. Establish a network for direct patient involvement. Cancer patients will be invited to join a national network with privacy safeguards. Patients will contribute data. Genetic profiles of their tumors will be derived and patients will be notified if their tumor profiles indicate that specific target treatments may be successful.
B. Clinical Trial network for immunotherapy will be established. Pediatric and adult patients could be recruited to trials. Immunotherapies could potentially include immunomodulatory antibodies, lymphocyte cell transfer, or vaccine therapy.
C. Develop ways to overcome resistance to therapy. Multidisciplinary teams will be established to study the biological mechanisms through which cancer cells are or become resistant to certain drugs.
D. Build a National Cancer Data Ecosystem. In this system, databases and data repositories will be generated for researchers, doctors and patients to share data on cancer.
E. Intensify research on major drivers of childhood cancer. Pediatric cancers are very frequently different from adult cancer in that they have fewer mutations. However, they also tend to have more chromosome and

gene rearrangements leading to generation of new proteins (oncoproteins). The panel noted that these fusion proteins possibly represent opportunities for development of target therapies.

F. Minimize cancer treatments' debilitating side effects. The panel noted that cancer treatments are frequently excruciating for patients. In addition, the short and long term side effects of cancer treatment are particularly alarming in children. The panel recommended research to address these issues.

G. Expand use of proven prevention and early detection. The panel emphasized the importance of preventative vaccination against human papilloma virus that causes cervical cancer, genital cancers and naso-pharyngeal cancer, and use of hepatitis B vaccine. Pre-symptomatic screening for tobacco-related cancers and for colorectal cancer should be increased. In addition, physicians and families should be aware of hereditary cancer syndromes and genetic testing for these should be carried out in individuals at risk. Hereditary cancer syndromes include breast ovarian cancer syndrome and specific forms of colorectal cancers.

H. Mine past patient data to predict future outcomes. The panel noted that much data on patients treated with conventional cancer therapy is available and tumor tissue is available. However, this data is not adequately mined to yield information on treatment efficacy or lack thereof.

I. Develop a 3D cancer atlas. Devise strategies to develop data on different regions in tumors and relationships of tumors to surrounding tissues and structures.

J. Develop new cancer technologies. These could include new diagnostic tools, also new tools for drug delivery, e.g. direct drug delivery into tumors.

Tumor Recurrences

Investigations are ongoing to determine factors that promote recurrences of tumor growth following apparently successful treatment. The HER2 gene encodes a specific receptor (human epidermal growth factor receptor 2). In approximately 25% of breast tumors, this receptor is over-expressed and this promotes tumor growth. Specific targeted therapy can be very successful in treating tumors with HER2 amplification. However, in some cases, tumors that were apparently eradicated, recur. Abravanel *et al.*

(2015) studied breast cancer tumors that were classified as HER2/Neu positive. They initially carried out studies in mouse models of this tumor. Their studies revealed that following apparently successful treatment, some tumor cells remained dormant in the breast. They determined that if the dormant tumor cells expressed a specific signaling molecule in the Notch pathway, they subsequently gave rise to new tumors. Abravanil then carried out a retrospective study of 4,000 cases of human breast cancer cases. They determined recurrences were more frequent in cases where tumors were positive for the NOTCH signaling molecules. They concluded that the use of inhibitors to downregulate Notch expression would reduce the incidence of relapses following HER2 targeted therapies.

Malladi et al. (2016) reported that a minority of disseminated cancer cells survived for years after removal of a tumor. They analyzed specific features of these cells and reported that that the cells often expressed the specific transcription factors SOX2 and SOX9. Furthermore, these cells expressed factors that silenced the WNT signaling pathway. These dormant cells suppressed cell division and they also evaded destruction in the immune system.

Tumor Heterogeneity and Therapy Resistance

It is important to emphasize that not all cells in a tumor are the same and that some cells may be more sensitive to therapy than other cells. All cells may therefore not be destroyed by the therapy or therapies used. It is also possible that tumor cells undergo continuous mutation processes and that specific mutations may promote resistance in a subset of cells. Processes that enable cancer cells to resist drugs include development of the capacity to inactivate a drug or capacity to transport a drug out of the cells. Specific tumor cells may also undergo changes in gene expression so that they are more efficient at repairing DNA damage caused by drugs. Alterations in gene expression may also allow cells to become more resistant to cell death (Housman et al., 2014).

New Approaches to Early Detection of Tumors

Since cancers are more successfully treated in the early stages than in later stages, there are ongoing intense studies to identify biomarkers that are present in the circulation or biomarkers that can be radiologically imaged in organs where tumors are located.

Radiopharmaceuticals are sometimes used to locate tumors radiologically. Radiopharmaceuticals may be radiolabeled antibodies to a specific protein known to be produced in high quantities by certain tumors. One example is a specific radiopharmaceutical used to detect pancreatic tumors. A specific protein, CA19-9 is over-produced by cancerous pancreatic cells and a radiopharmaceutical compound has been produced and is in clinical trials for detection of pancreatic tumors (SK website) (https://www. mskcc.org/search?keys=CA19-9+).

New Approaches to Clinical Trials

The early stages of clinical trials involve specific tests to ascertain the safety of a particular compound to be used as therapy. Later stages involve ascertainment of the capacity of a therapeutic agent to eliminate disease or significantly reduce the deleterious manifestations of a disease.

Historically, clinical trials were designed as prospective randomized double arm trials. If clinically affected individuals were included in a trial in one arm of the trial, the patients received a specific medication and patients in the other arm of the trial did not receive the medication (Hohl, 2015).

Traditionally, clinical trials each focused on a specific type of cancer classified on clinical and histopathological measures.

New trial designs have been developed for targeted therapies in cancer. Basket trials target a specific gene mutation that occurs in different types of tumors. All tumors that harbor that specific gene mutation are treated with a specific targeting drug.

Umbrella trials involve the testing of different drugs on the different mutations that are present in a specific tumor type.

Another important advance in clinical trials has been the initiation of adaptive trials. In adaptive trials, data is analyzed not only at the end of the trial. Data is analyzed at different stages of a trial and alterations in the trial procedures can be made based on information yielded by the early analysis. For example, if a group of patients are not improving on a certain medication or with a specific medication dose whereas another group of patients with the same disorder or the same mutation are improving on a particular medication or dosage, the medication or dosage can be changed for the first group of patients who were not improving. Bayesian analysis is used in statistical studies for adaptive clinical trials (Berry, 2015). In Bayesian analysis, it is possible to update the probability of a hypothesis as more information becomes available.

47 Improved Health, Prolonged Survival and Wellness

In many countries in the world, health and well-being have increased significantly over the past several decades. Are these improvements due to improved living conditions or due to improved healthcare? The answer I believe is that both are important.

The Wellness Concept

In 1991, Emory Cowen published an article entitled "In pursuit of Wellness". In that article, he dealt largely with psychological wellness and he also promoted the concept of "building health rather than fighting disease".

Cowen proposed four key concepts in pursuing the Wellness objective. These included enhancing competence, resilience, empowerment of individuals and modification of the social system. He realized that competence clearly differs at different ages and life stages; in children it had to do with school, later it had to do with work skills. He also emphasized competency in interpersonal communication, problem solving, assertiveness and in anger management.

With respect to resilience, Cowen noted that some children raised in disadvantageous situations manifested remarkable resilience that facilitated their later adaptations and accomplishments. He promoted studies to analyze resilience.

Cowen stressed that empowerment is a value, particularly when it is accompanied by competency. Wellness would be promoted by empowerment and competency, but wellness would be negatively impacted when empowerment and competencies were not matched.

Over the past few decades, several organizations have documented dimensions of Wellness. Wellness has come to imply physical health, adequate nutrition, as well as social, emotional, occupational and intellectual wellness.

Seven dimensions, proposed by University of California, Riverside, also include environmental wellness and responsibility to positively impact one's environment. Occupational wellness in their statement includes the concept of making a positive impact through work efforts. Intellectual wellness includes the desire to learn new concepts and to be open to new ideas Spiritual wellness encompasses the ability to establish peace and harmony in life: https://wellness.ucr.edu/seven_dimensions.html.

In the 21st century however, we remain confronted by the extreme complexity of a number of late onset chronic diseases. Particularly challenging are the late onset neurodegenerative diseases, Alzheimer's disease, Parkinson's disease and amyotrophic lateral sclerosis. Cancer remains a problem; however, hope for a cure seems more alive there.

Again I turn to Lewis Thomas (1977):

"The plain fact of the matter is that we do not know enough facts of the matter and we should be more open about our ignorance".

In an essay entitled 'The medical lessons from History' written in 1977, Thomas also noted: "an undercurrent of almost outrageous optimism about what may lie ahead for the treatment of human disease if we can only keep learning".

48 Health: Human and Planetary

Expanding Concepts of Health and of the Dimensions of Environmental Impact

In 1948, the World Health Organization defined human health as: "A state of complete physical, mental and social well-being and not merely the absence of disease and infirmity."

The European Union Strategy on Environment and Health (2003) recognized that poverty and social factors are the main determinants of human health and they recognized that environmental factors play important roles.

From my early years of training I became acutely aware of the links between poor health and poverty, social factors, and degraded living conditions. These links continue to be readily recognizable in many places in the world. Sadly, the abilities of an individual citizen to turn these conditions around remain restricted. Turn arounds require the collective will and actions of society and of citizens at many different levels.

Perhaps I turned away from problems that seemed impossible for me to solve. Over the course of many years, I have worked to understand genetic and genomic factors and to determine their roles in the causation of human disease. When I embarked on a career in human genetics, it seemed that this was an important subject to which time and energy should be devoted. In the early nineteen sixties, relatively little was known about the underlying molecular defects that led to birth defects and inborn errors of metabolism.

A few years ago, a biologist who was visiting the university where I work asked to visit with me because of my involvement with studies of human genetic variation. As we ended our meeting he made a remark that stopped me in my tracks and stayed with me. He said "Of course we should rather be studying variation in plants, birds, insects and four-legged animals before they all disappear. Humans are a bane upon the earth". Contemplating his statement, I began to question if, in working toward the promotion of human health, I have in fact worked toward destruction of the earth.

Our lives are filled with accounts of loss of habitats and loss of species that have sustained man physically and spiritually over eons. At times, a sense of helplessness floods in. The trajectory that mankind is following seems destined to end in disaster.

Progress in our understanding of biology and genetics has led us to understand how similar all life forms on earth are in terms of their metabolism and the building blocks of their genetic material. Many of the poisons we designed to damage other life forms turn out to be damaging to humans. Exposure to such poisons need not be continuous to cause damage. Even short-term exposure can be harmful to the developing fetus.

However, I cannot remain suffused with this negativism and sense of hopelessness for long. I answer a resounding "Yes!" to the question: "Is it possible to be a humanist and an environmentalist?" Being a humanist means believing that people matter, that they have a right to physical and spiritual nurture. It means that working toward freedom from want and disease, we consider needs of both body and spirit. For optimal health, people do not only require a food supply and shelter, they require that there be a healthy environment and that there be wilderness and biodiversity. I have to proceed with faith that given sufficient education and opportunity, most people will make good decisions for their families and their communities. I realize, too, the important roles that ongoing discussions of ethics, psychology, philosophy and the arts will play as we work to resolve problems and develop solutions.

In 1949, Aldo Leopold's influential book *A Sand County Almanac* was published. His description of the natural world and its creatures reawaken the sense of wonder and inspire. In addition, Leopold addressed ethics that lay the groundwork for conservation. He wrote: "That land is a community is the basic concept of Ecology, but that land is to be loved and respected is an extension of Ethics".

Planetary Health

From Wendell Berry (1969): "We have lived our lives by the assumption that what was good for us would be good for the world. We have been wrong. We must change our lives so that it will be possible to live by the contrary assumption, what is good for the world will be good for us. And that requires that we make the effort to know the world and learn what is good for it."

Major reports on planetary health and its relation to human health published in recent decades include the Millennium ecosystems assessment (2003) and the Rockefeller Foundation–Lancet Commission report (Whitmee et al., 2015). These reports emphasized the degree to which humans are dependent upon healthy ecosystems. Key factors implicated in environmental change include over-consumption, over-use of resources and population growth.

The Millennium ecosystems assessment concluded that "the ability of the planet's ecosystems to sustain future generations cannot be taken for granted".

A key concept emphasized in the Rockefeller Foundation–Lancet Commission on Planetary Health report is that human health and civilization are dependent upon flourishing natural systems. They urged: "Promotion of sustainable and equitable patterns of consumption, reducing population growth and harnessing the power of technology for change". The commission urged creation of integrated surveillance to collect health, socioeconomic and environmental data, and also communication of risk data to policy makers and to the public.

The commission report emphasized that improvements in health and reduction of poverty over the past century have been supported by the Earth's ecological and biophysical systems. They stated, however, that we have now entered the Anthropocene epoch. This is defined as the epoch when human activities have substantial global effects on Earth systems.

These reports discussed key variables to be measured in reviewing global systems under pressure including analysis of climate change, stratospheric ozone depletion, atmospheric aerosol loading, ocean acidification, usage of available fresh water including ground water, land system changes and biosphere integrity and biogeochemical flows. Biogeochemical flows involve addition of nitrogen and phosphorus to run off, e.g. from excess fertilizer use, their accumulation in water, excess growth of algae and depletion of oxygen in water. Land system changes include loss of forest.

Increases in atmospheric concentrations of carbon dioxide, methane, nitrous oxide and black carbon contribute to climate change. Biosphere integrity is compromised by chemical pollution. The commission noted that this derives from agriculture, from mining, production that uses solvents and other chemicals, and from drug and pharmaceutical pollution. An important factor to consider is how health systems impact the environment.

Reduction in available fresh water impairs access to safe drinking water. Reduction in water also leads to impaired sanitation and results in a significant increase in the incidence of diarrhea in some parts of the world.

River fragmentation and eutrophication of fresh water promotes increases in the number of snails in water and this contributes to schistosomiasis.

The Rockefeller Foundation–Lancet report noted that under-nutrition leading to impaired physical and cognitive development still impacts 1 in 4 of the world's children under five years of age. This problem is exacerbated in areas where agricultural productivity has been reduced, in part due to soil nutrient depletion and climate change.

It is important to factor in food waste. It is estimated that 30–50% of food produced is wasted. Waste may be connected to defects in harvesting of food, in storage of food, in transportation, marketing or in consumption. It is also important to note that over-nutrition also constitutes an important problem. Over-nutrition constitutes a risk factor for specific non-communicable diseases. Diets with high content of animal proteins require increased land usage. The Rockefeller Foundation–Lancet commission report emphasized the importance of promoting healthy low environmental impact diets. The greenhouse gas accumulation associated with production of one gram of animal protein was estimated to be 250 times higher than that required for production of one gram of plant-derived protein.

WHO reports indicate that non-communicable diseases, including cardiovascular diseases, diabetes, cancer and chronic respiratory diseases, lead to 14 million premature deaths annually in the world. Premature deaths are described as death before the age of 70 years. The reports note that premature deaths are often linked to risk factors that include lack of physical activity, tobacco use and harmful use of alcohol.

Degraded forest habitats likely contribute to the transmission of zoonotic diseases.

ARBO viruses

ARBO is an acronym for arthropod-borne viruses. The arthropods that carry these viruses are primarily mosquitoes and ticks but also tsetse flies, black flies and fleas. In recent years, infections due to ARBO viruses have been increasing in many parts of the world. There have been significant increases in the territories infested with mosquitoes in recent decades. This is attributed in part to loss of forests but is largely attributed to increased urbanization. Of particular concern are urban areas where standing water accumulates close to homes. Some writers have also drawn attention to mosquito breeding that occurs in dumps of old tires (http.//www.epa.illinois.gov/topics/waste-management/waste-disposal/used-tires/mosquito-borne-illnesses/index).

The WHO emphasizes that the worldwide distribution of ARBO viral-related diseases has been influenced by increases in global travel and trade, by unplanned urbanization and environmental challenges, including climate change.

Two types of mosquitoes are of particular concern, *Aedes aegypti* and *Aedes albopictus*. Kraemer *et al.* (2015) reported that *Aedes aegypti* occurs in large areas of the tropics and in sub-tropical regions north and south of the equator. They also occur in Madagascar, India, South-East Asia and in the northern coastal regions of Australia. *Aedes aegypti* mosquitoes also occur in the Americas, in Brazil in particular and to a lesser degree in Venezuela and Mexico. In the USA, *Aedes aegypti* occurs in Florida and in the adjacent coastal regions. In Europe, they occur particularly in Italy.

The distribution of *Aedes albopictus* is similar to that of *Aedes aegypti*. However, *Aedes albopictus* distribution extends further into southern Europe and it also extends also extends further into the south-eastern regions of the USA. *Aedes albopictus* has also been found in China and Japan. *Culex* mosquitoes also transmit specific ARBO viral diseases.

Fauci and Morens (2016) reported that ARBO viruses are predominantly RNA viruses. They often have complex life cycles that include mammals or sometimes birds. There is evidence that ARBO viruses have been transmitted to domestic animals including horses and pigs. In addition, there is now evidence that additional types of mosquitoes transmit ARBO viruses.

Diseases Caused by ARBO Viruses

The best known disease transmitted by *Aedes aegypti* is yellow fever. Other *Aedes aegypti* transmitted diseases include Dengue, Chikungunya and Rift valley fevers and most recently, Zika virus infections. Dengue fever is listed by the WHO as the fastest growing ARBO viral diseases (Kraemer *et al.*, 2015). The WHO report noted that ARBO viral diseases include Dengue Fever, Chikungunja and West Nile viral disease.

Ticks transmit ARBO viruses that cause Congo hemorrhagic fever, Lyme disease relapsing fever, Tick-borne encephalitis; they also transmit Rickettsial diseases. Tsetse flies transmit trypanosomiases. Fleas transmit plague and Rickettsial diseases. Black flies transmit river blindness, also known as onchocerciasis.

Zika ARBO virus

Fauci and Morens (2016) reviewed the emergence of Zika virus. They noted that Zika virus was first discovered in the Zika forest in Uganda in 1947, in studies on primates and mosquitoes. African researchers also reported that Zika virus epidemics tended to follow Chikungunya epizootic infections or human epidemics. Following the initial description of these epidemics, the viruses then spread west and east. By 2015, Zika virus or Zika virus antibodies were found in South America particularly in Brazil, Mexico and Puerto Rica, and also in India, South-East Asia and Polynesia.

Fauci and Morens reported that Zika virus infections are most commonly described as mild disorders associated with rash, fever and joint pains. However, in French Polynesia during a Zika virus epidemic there were also cases of Zika virus infection that developed neurological complications sometimes diagnosed as Guillain–Barre syndrome with manifestation of peripheral paralysis.

In Brazil, occurrence of cases of microcephaly born to women who had Zika virus infections during pregnancy has raised alarms. Fauci and Morens noted that intensive investigations are required to determine the possible connection between Zika virus and microcephaly. They noted further that PCR-based gene tests were available, but that test could not always accurately distinguish between Chikungunya viral infection and Zika virus infection.

Fauci and Morens emphasized that broad spectrum anti-viral antibiotics were urgently needed. In addition, vaccines were urgently needed. Ideally, vaccines and vaccine platforms would be able to be readily modified as new viral antigens emerged. In November 2016, a report from NIH revealed that a vaccine to protect against Zika virus infections is in Phase II clinical trials.

Convergence

In a 2014 editorial in Science magazine, Sharp and Leshner wrote: "Every major challenge of modern life, such as ensuring energy, health, and water and food security in a sustainable world with a predicted nine billion inhabitants has complex science and technology components". They stressed that convergent approaches to solutions are required. These solutions would require integration of knowledge from life, physical, social and economic sciences and from engineering.

There is growing agreement that solving of significant world societal and health problems will require convergence of the expertise of different disciplines. Convergence in this instance can be defined as the coming together of insights and approaches from originally distinct fields. Problems that would benefit from the attention of convergent disciplines include the need for secure food supplies, for efficient energy production and development of more effective treatments to combat the high costs of inefficient treatments.

A report from the USA National Academy of Sciences (NAS) (2015) emphasized that because convergence relies on integrating expertise from multiple fields and multiple partners "an open and inclusive culture, a common set of concepts and metrics and shared sets of institutional and research goals are required".

The authors of the NAS report recognized that scientific advances comprise the combination of results from incremental advances in knowledge as well as significant breakthroughs.

References

Abravanel DL, Belka GK, Pan TC, et al. (2015). Notch promotes recurrence of dormant tumor cells following HER2/neu-targeted therapy. J Clin Invest 125(6):2484–96. doi: 10.1172/JCI74883. PMID:25961456.

Bavle, AA, Lin FY, Parsons DW. (2016). Applications of genomic sequencing in pediatric CNS tumors. *Oncology (Williston Park)* **30(5):**411–23. PMID:27188671.

Berry DA. (2016). Emerging innovations in clinical trial design. *Clin Pharmacol Ther* **99(1):**82–91. doi: 10.1002/cpt.285. PMID:26561040.

Berry W. (1969). *The Long-legged house.* Harcourt, Brace, Jovanovich; New York.

Bianco P, Cao X, Frenette PS, *et al.* (2013). The meaning, the sense and the significance: translating the science of mesenchymal stem cells into medicine. *Nat Med* **19(1):**35–42. doi: 10.1038/nm.3028. PMID:23296015.

Blackburn EH, Greider CW, Szostak JW. (2006). Telomeres and telomerase: the path from maize, Tetrahymena and yeast to human cancer and aging. *Nat Med* **12(10):**1133–8. PMID:17024208.

Board on Life Sciences USA National Academy of Sciences (NAS) (2015). Convergence: facilitating transdisciplinary integration of life sciences, physical sciences, engineering, and beyond (2014). Available online at: https://www.nap.edu/download/18722.

Chen L, Han X. (2015). Anti-PD-1/PD-L1 therapy of human cancer: past, present, and future. *J Clin Invest* **125(9):**3384–91. doi: 10.1172/JCI80011. PMID:26325035.

Cheung KJ, Ewald AJ. (2016). A collective route to metastasis: seeding by tumor cell clusters. *Science* **352(6282):**167–9. doi: 10.1126/science.aaf6546. PMID:27124449.

Cowen EL. (1991). In pursuit of wellness. *Am Psychol* **46(4):**404–408. http://dx.doi.org/10.1037/0003-066X.46.4.404.

Dijkstra KK, Voabil P, Schumacher TN, Voest EE. (2016). Genomics — and transcriptomics-based patient selection for cancer treatment with immune checkpoint inhibitors: A review. *JAMA Oncol* **2(11):**1490–1495. doi: 10.1001/jamaoncol.2016.2214. PMID:27491050.

Esch MB, Smith AS, Prot JM, *et al.* (2014). How multi-organ microdevices can help foster drug development. *Adv Drug Deliv Rev* **69–70:**158–69. doi: 10.1016/j.addr.2013.12.003. PMID:24412641.

European Union Strategy on Environment and Health (2003). http://ec.europa.eu/health/healthy_environments/policy/health_environment/strategy_en.htm

Evans MJ, Kaufman MH. (1981). Establishment in culture of pluripotential cells from mouse embryos. *Nature* **292(5819):**154–6. PMID:7242681.

Fauci AS, Morens DM. (2016). Zika virus in the Americas--yet another Arbovirus threat. *N Engl J Med* **374(7):**601–4. doi: 10.1056/NEJMp1600297. PMID:26761185.

Fesnak AD, June CH, Levine BL. (2016). Engineered T cells: the promise and challenges of cancer immunotherapy. *Nat Rev Cancer* **16(9):**566–81. doi: 10.1038/nrc.2016.97. PMID:27550819.

Freeman GJ, Long AJ, Iwai Y, *et al.* (2000). Engagement of the PD-1 immunoinhibitory receptor by a novel B7 family member leads to negative regulation of lymphocyte activation. *J Exp Med* **192(7):**1027–34. PMID:11015443.

Funakoshi S, Miki K, Takaki T *et al.* (2016). Enhanced engraftment, proliferation, and therapeutic potential in heart using optimized human iPSC-derived cardiomyocytes. *Sci Rep* **6:**19111. doi: 10.1038/srep19111. PMID:26743035.

Gurdon JB. (1962). Adult frogs derived from the nuclei of single somatic cells. *Dev Biol* **4:**256–73. PMID:13903027.

Gurdon J. (2009). Nuclear reprogramming in eggs. *Nat Med* **15(10):**1141–4. doi: 10.1038/nm1009-1141. PMID:19812574.

Haché M, Swoboda KJ, Sethna N, *et al.* (2016). Intrathecal Injections in children with spinal muscular atrophy: nusinersen clinical trial experience. *J Child Neurol* **31(7):**899–906. doi: 10.1177/0883073815627882. PMID:26823478.

Hayflick L, Moorhead PS. (1961). The serial cultivation of human diploid cell strains. *Exp Cell Res* **25**:585–621. PMID:13905658.

Hockemeyer D, Jaenisch R. (2016). Induced pluripotent stem cells meet genome editing. *Cell Stem Cell* **18(5):**573–86. doi: 10.1016/j.stem.2016.04.013. PMID:27152442.

Hofman P, Popper HH. (2016). Pathologists and liquid biopsies: to be or not to be? *Virchows Arch* **469(6):**601–609. PMID:27553354.

Hohl RJ. (2015). Oncology trial design: more accurately and efficiently advancing the field. *Clin Pharmacol Ther* **97(5):**430–2. doi: 10.1002/cpt.94. PMID:25684240.

Hoshino A, Costa-Silva B, Lyden D, *et al.* (2015). Tumour exosome integrins determine organotropic metastasis. *Nature* **527(7578):**329–35. doi: 10.1038/nature15756. PMID:26524530.

Housman G, Byler S, Heerboth S, *et al.* (2014). Drug resistance in cancer: an overview. *Cancers (Basel)* **6(3):**1769–92. doi: 10.3390/cancers6031769. PMID:25198391.

Kleinsmith LJ, Pierce GB Jr. Multipotentiality of single embryonal carcinoma cells. *Cancer Res* **24:**1544–51. PMID:14234000.

Kranz LM, Diken M, Haas H, *et al.* (2016). Systemic RNA delivery to dendritic cells exploits antiviral defence for cancer immunotherapy. *Nature* **534(7607):**396–401. doi: 10.1038/nature18300. PMID:27281205.

Kraemer MU, Sinka ME, Duda KA, *et al.* (2015). The global distribution of the arbovirus vectors *Aedes aegypti* and *Ae. albopictus*. *Elife* **4:** e08347. doi: 10.7554/eLife.08347. PMID:26126267.

Kuilman T, Michaloglou C, Mooi WJ, Peeper DS. (2010). The essence of senescence. *Gene Dev* **24(22):**2463–79. Doi: 10.1101/gad.1971610. PMID:21078816.

Lapasset L, Milhavet O, Prieur A, et al. (2011). Rejuvenating senescent and centenarian human cells by reprogramming through the pluripotent state. Genes Dev 25(21):2248–53. doi: 10.1101/gad.173922.111. PMID:22056670.

Leach DR, Krummel MF, Allison JP. (1996). Enhancement of antitumor immunity by CTLA-4 blockade. Science 271(5256):1734–6. PMID:8596936.

Lemey C, Milhavet O, Lemaitre JM. (2015). iPSCs as a major opportunity to understand and cure age-related diseases. Biogerontology 16(4):399–410. doi: 10.1007/s10522-015-9579-7. PMID:25981448.

Leopold A. (1949). Sand County Almanac. Published by Oxford University Press.

López-Otín C, Blasco MA, Partridge L, et al. (2013) The hallmarks of aging. Cell 153(6):1194–217. doi: 10.1016/j.cell.2013.05.039. PMID:23746838.

Maeder ML, Gersbach CA. (2016). Genome-editing technologies for gene and cell therapy. Mol Ther 24(3):430–46. doi: 10.1038/mt.2016.10. PMID:26755333.

Malladi S, Macalinao DG, Jin X, et al. (2016). Metastatic latency and immune evasion through autocrine inhibition of WNT. Cell 165(1):45–60. doi: 10.1016/j.cell.2016.02.025. PMID:27015306.

Martin GR, Evans MJ. (1974). The morphology and growth of a pluripotent teratocarcinoma cell line and its derivatives in tissue culture. Cell 2(3): 163–72. PMID:4416368.

Martin GR, Evans MJ. (1975). Differentiation of clonal lines of teratocarcinoma cells: formation of embryoid bodies in vitro. Proc Natl Acad Sci USA 72(4):1441–5. PMID:1055416.

Martin GR. (1981). Isolation of a pluripotent cell line from early mouse embryos cultured in medium conditioned by teratocarcinoma stem cells. Proc Natl Acad Sci USA 78(12):7634–8. PMID:6950406.

Martin OA, Anderson RL, Narayan K, MacManus MP. (2016). Does the mobilization of circulating tumour cells during cancer therapy cause metastasis? Nat Rev Clin Oncol [Epub ahead of print]. doi: 10.1038/nrclinonc.2016.128. PMID:27550857.

McNeish J, Gardner JP, Wainger BJ, et al. (2015). From dish to bedside: lessons learned while translating findings from a stem cell model of disease to a clinical trial. Cell Stem Cell 17(1):8–10. doi: 10.1016/j.stem.2015.06.013. PMID:26140603.

Melo SA, Luecke LB, Kahlert C, et al. (2015). Glypican-1 identifies cancer exosomes and detects early pancreatic cancer. Nature 523(7559):177–82. doi: 10.1038/nature14581. PMID:26106858.

Millennium ecosystem assessment: http://www.millenniumassessment.org/en/index.html.

NIH Zika virus vaccine: https://www.nih.gov/news-events/news-releases/nih-begins-testing-investigational-zika-vaccine-humans.

Pan W, Gu W, Nagpal S, *et al.* (2015). Brain tumor mutations detected in cerebral spinal fluid. *Clin Chem* **61(3):**514–22. doi: 10.1373/clinchem.2014.235457.

Park CY, Kim DH, Son JS, *et al.* (2015). Functional correction of large factor VIII gene chromosomal inversions in hemophilia A patient-derived iPSCs using CRISPR-Cas9. *Cell Stem Cell* **17(2):**213–20. doi: 10.1016/j.stem.2015.07.001. PMID:26212079.

Reardon S. (2016). First CRISPR clinical trial gets green light from US panel. The technique's first test in people could begin as early as the end of the year. *Nature News* 22 June 2016.

Rosenberg SA, Restifo NP. (2015). Adoptive cell transfer as personalized immunotherapy for human cancer. *Science* **348(6230):**62–8. doi: 10.1126/science. aaa4967. PMID:25838374.

Ross SB, Fraser ST, Semsarian C. (2016). Induced pluripotent stem cells in the inherited cardiomyopathies: from disease mechanisms to novel therapies. *Trends Cardiovasc Med* **26(8):**663–672. doi: 10.1016/j.tcm.2016.05.001. PMID:27296521.

Sander JD, Joung JK. (2014). CRISPR-Cas systems for editing, regulating and targeting genomes. *Nat Biotechnol* **32(4):**347–55. doi: 10.1038/nbt.2842. PMID:24584096.

Sharp PA, Leshner AI. (2014). Meeting global challenges. *Science* **343(6171):**579. doi: 10.1126/science.1250725. PMID:24503818.

Siravegna G, Mussolin B, Buscarino M, *et al.* (2015). Clonal evolution and resistance to EGFR blockade in the blood of colorectal cancer patients. *Nat Med* **21(7):**795–801. doi: 10.1038/nm.3870. PMID:26030179.

Sullivan LB, Gui DY, Heiden MG. (2016). Altered metabolite levels in cancer: implications for tumour biology and cancer therapy. *Nat Rev Cancer* **16(11):** 680–693. doi: 10.1038/nrc.2016.85. PMID:27658530.

Takahashi K, Yamanaka S. (2006). Induction of pluripotent stem cells from mouse embryonic and adult fibroblast cultures by defined factors. *Cell* **126(4):** 663–76. PMID:16904174.

Takahashi K, Yamanaka S. (2016). A decade of transcription factor-mediated reprogramming to pluripotency. *Nat Rev Mol Cell Biol* **17(3):**183–93. doi: 10.1038/nrm.2016.8. PMID:26883003.

Thomas L. (1977). *The medical lessons of history.* First Published in Daedalus Journal of American Academy of Arts and Sciences, Boston. Reproduced in: *A Long Line of Cells.* (1990) Published by Book of the Month Club. Quotation is on p. 218.

Thomas L. (1977). The technology of medicine. In: Thomas L. *The Lives of the Cell.* Re-published in 1997, The Viking Press.

Thomson JA, Itskovitz-Eldor J, Shapiro SS, *et al.* (1998). Embryonic stem cell lines derived from human blastocysts. *Science* **282(5391):**1145–7. Erratum in: *Science* **282(5395):**1827 (1998). PMID:9804556.

Topalian SL, Hodi FS, Brahmer J.R (2012). Safety, activity and immune correlates of anti-PD-1 antibody in cancer. *N Engl J Med* **366(26)**; 2443–54. doi:10.1056/ NEJMoa1200690.PMID: 22658127.

Trounson A, DeWitt ND. (2016). Pluripotent stem cells progressing to the clinic. *Nat Rev Mol Cell Biol* **17(3).**194–200. doi: 10.1038/nrm.2016.10. PMID:26908143.

Traxler EA, Yao Y, Wang YD, *et al.* (2016). A genome-editing strategy to treat β-hemoglobinopathies that recapitulates a mutation associated with a benign genetic condition. *Nat Med* **22(9):**987–90. doi: 10.1038/nm.4170. PMID:27525524.

Wagner JE Jr, Brunstein CG, Boitano AE, *et al.* (2016). Phase I/II Trial of StemRegenin-1 expanded umbilical cord blood hematopoietic stem cells supports testing as a stand-alone graft. *Cell Stem Cell* **18(1):**144–55. doi: 10.1016/j.stem.2015.10.004. PMID:26669897.

Wang Y, Springer S, Zhang M, *et al.* (2015). Detection of tumor-derived DNA in cerebrospinal fluid of patients with primary tumors of the brain and spinal cord. *Proc Natl Acad Sci USA* **112(31):**9704–9. doi: 10.1073/pnas.1511694112. PMID:26195750.

Wainger BJ, Kiskinis E, Mellin C, *et al.* (2014). Intrinsic membrane hyperexcitability of amyotrophic lateral sclerosis patient-derived motor neurons. *Cell Rep* **7(1):** 1–11. doi: 10.1016/j.celrep.2014.03.019. PMID:24703839.

Whitmee S, Haines A, Beyrer C, *et al.* (2015). Safeguarding human health in the Anthropocene epoch: report of the rockefeller foundation-lancet commission on planetary health. *Lancet* **386(10007):**1973–2028. doi 10.1016/S0140-6736 (15)60901-1. PMID:26188744.

World Health Organization (1948). http://www.who.int/about/definition/en/print. html

WHO Global status report on noncommunicable diseases 2014: www.who.int/ nmh/publications/ncd-status-report-2014/en.

Ye L, Wang J, Tan Y, *et al.* (2016). Genome editing using CRISPR-Cas9 to create the HPFH genotype in HSPCs: an approach for treating sickle cell disease and β-thalassemia. *Proc Natl Acad Sci USA* **113(38):**10661–5. doi: 10.1073/ pnas.1612075113. PMID:27601644.

Yu J, Vodyanik MA, Thomson JA, *et al.* (2007). Induced pluripotent stem cell lines derived from human somatic cells. *Science* **318(5858):**1917–20. PMID:18029452.

Index

Printed in the United States
By Bookmasters